W0080581

Lasers in
Operative Dentistry
and Endodontics

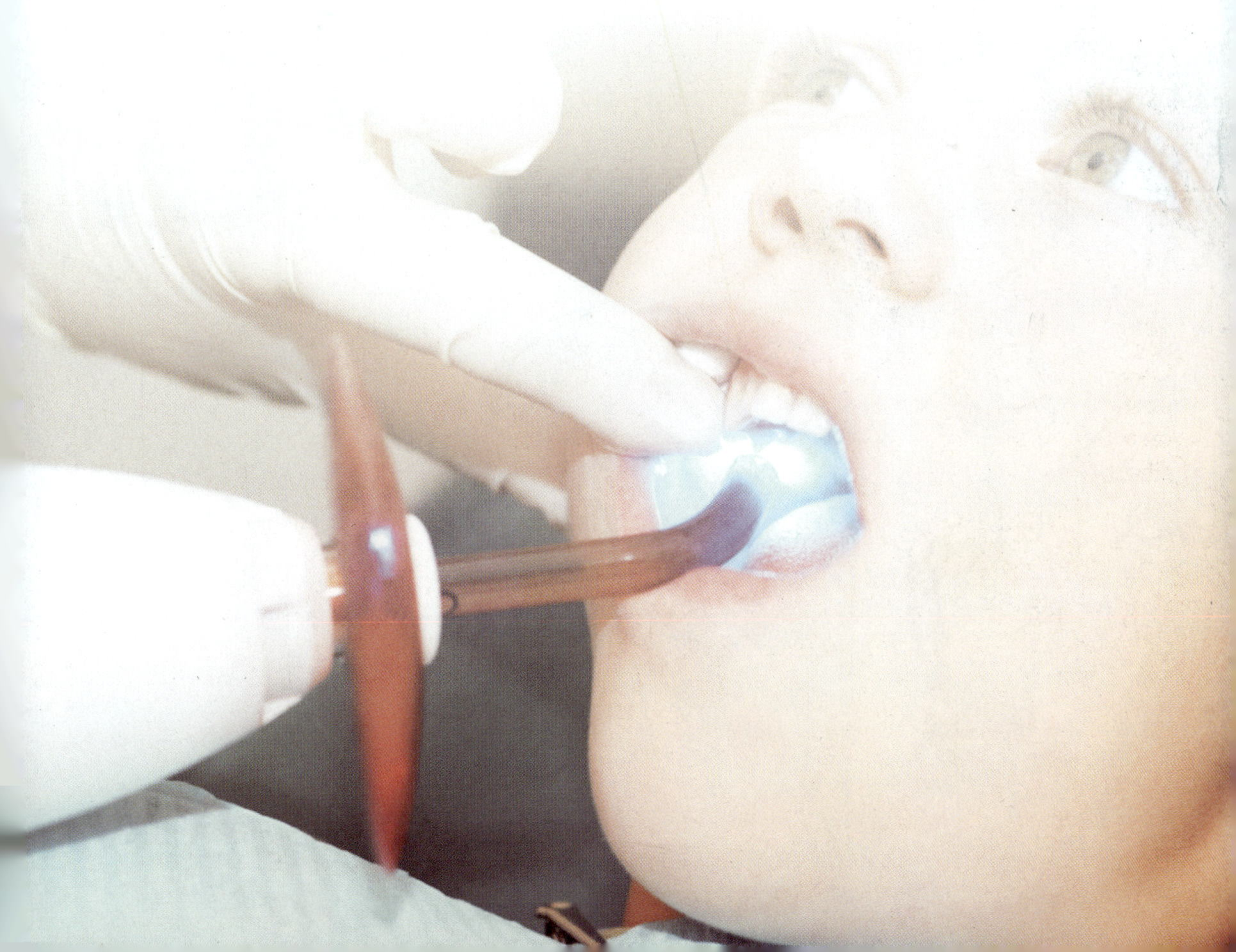

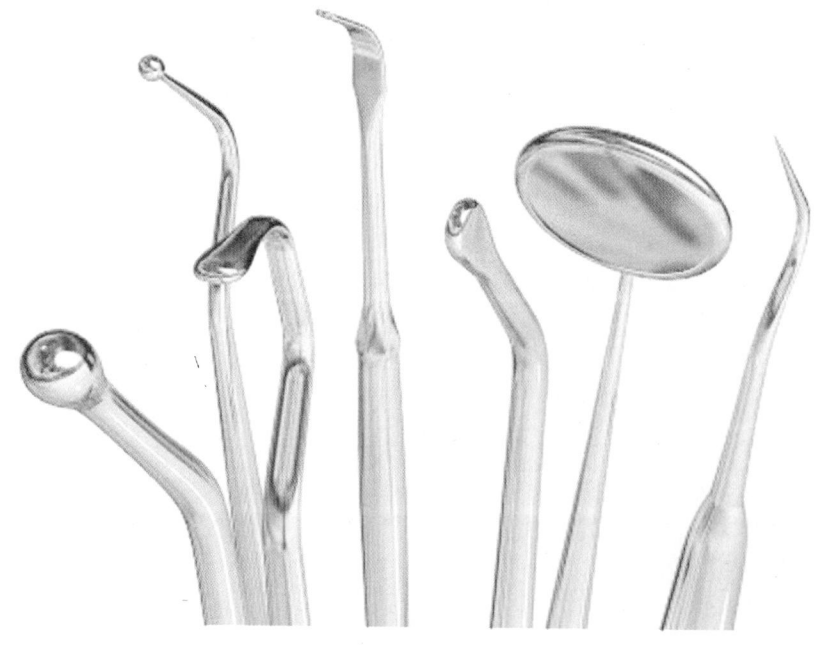

Lasers in Operative Dentistry and Endodontics

Vinisha Pandey
MDS (Conservative Dentistry and Endodontics)

Assistant Professor
Department of Conservative Dentistry
Rama Dental College
Kanpur, UP

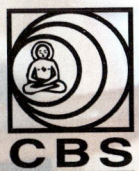

CBS

CBS Publishers & Distributors Pvt Ltd

New Delhi • Bengaluru • Chennai • Kochi • Mumbai • Pune
Hyderabad • Kolkata • Nagpur • Patna • Vijayawada

Disclaimer

Science and technology are constantly changing fields. New research and experience broaden the scope of information and knowledge. The author has tried her best in giving information available to her while preparing the material for this book. Although, all efforts have been made to ensure optimum accuracy of the material, yet it is quite possible some errors might have been left uncorrected. The publisher, the printer and the author will not be held responsible for any inadvertent errors, omissions or inaccuracies.

Lasers in Operative Dentistry and Endodontics

ISBN: 978-81-239-2521-9

Copyright © Author and Publisher

First Edition: 2015

All rights reserved. No part of this book may be reproduced or transmitted in any form or by any means, electronic or mechanical, including photocopying, recording, or any information storage and retrieval system without permission, in writing, from the author and the publisher.

Published by Satish Kumar Jain and produced by Varun Jain for

CBS Publishers & Distributors Pvt Ltd

4819/XI Prahlad Street, 24 Ansari Road, Daryaganj, New Delhi 110 002, India.

Ph: 23289259, 23266861, 23266867   Fax: 011-23243014   Website: www.cbspd.com
e-mail: delhi@cbspd.com; cbspubs@airtelmail.in

Corporate Office: 204 FIE, Industrial Area, Patparganj, Delhi 110 092

Ph: 4934 4934   Fax: 4934 4935   e-mail: publishing@cbspd.com; publicity@cbspd.com

Branches

- **Bengaluru:** Seema House 2975, 17th Cross, K.R. Road,
  Banasankari 2nd Stage, Bengaluru 560 070, Karnataka
  Ph: +91-80-26771678/79   Fax: +91-80-26771680   e-mail: bangalore@cbspd.com
- **Chennai:** 20, West Park Road, Shenoy Nagar, Chennai 600 030, Tamil Nadu
  Ph: +91-44-26260666, 26208620   Fax: +91-44-42032115   e-mail: chennai@cbspd.com
- **Kochi:** 36/14 Kalluvilakam, Lissie Hospital Road, Kochi 682 018, Kerala
  Ph: +91-484-4059061-65   Fax: +91-484-4059065   e-mail: kochi@cbspd.com
- **Mumbai:** 83-C, Dr E Moses Road, Worli, Mumbai-400018, Maharashtra
  Ph: +91-22-24902340/41   Fax: +91-22-24902342   e-mail: mumbai@cbspd.com
- **Pune:** Bhuruk Prestige, Sr. No. 52/12/2+1+3/2 Narhe, Haveli
  (Near Katraj-Dehu Road Bypass), Pune 411 041, Maharashtra
  Ph: +91-20-64704058, 64704059, 32392277 Fax: +91-20-24300160   e-mail: pune@cbspd.com

Representatives

- **Hyderabad**   0-9885175004   • **Kolkata**   0-9831437309, 0-9051152362
- **Nagpur**   0-9021734563   • **Patna**   0-9334159340   • **Vijayawada**   0-9000660880

Printed at: HT Media Ltd., Noida

to
_____

my loving parents
whose cherished blessings are behind
whatever success I have achieved in life. They have guided me and
helped me to lead the journey to clinical perfection

my husband
for his support and for making my life more meaningful

my brother
for always being there when I needed him.

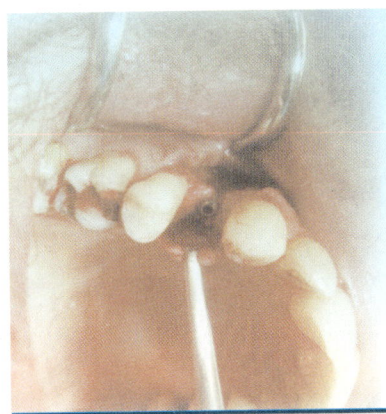

Foreword

It is my pleasure and honor to write the the the Foreword to this book by *Dr Vinisha Pandey*. As a general dentist who was a pioneer in bringing lasers into my practice, I very much appreciate the contents of this work. The text presents both the fundamental principles of laser operation and the many clinical applications of this amazing technology. There are wonderful details explaining concepts such as interaction of laser energy with specific dental tissue compounds as well as how the different available wavelengths can be utilized. Various dental procedures can be performed with dental lasers, and Dr Pandey discusses the advantages and the protocols.

Dental lasers were first introduced about 25 years ago, and this book reflects very current information. I am confident that the reader will easily be able to appreciate how these instruments can provide better dental care for our patients. Equally important is the fact that dental laser practitioners can have renewed confidence in their clinical treatments, knowing that they are more precise in targeting disease while being more conservative in protecting healthy dental structures.

I hope you find the book both educational and inspirational.

Donald J. Coluzzi DDS

Donald J. Coluzzi, DDS
Health Science Clinical Professor
University of California, San Francisco
School of Dentistry

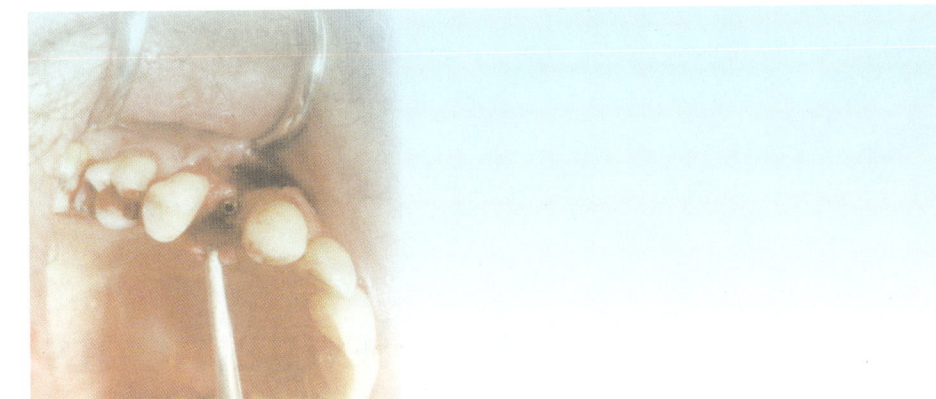

Preface

Lasers in operative dentistry and endodontics have been termed as the latest inventions in the recent paradigm of dentistry. Light has always astonished man and this book has been written to amplify arguably the best and most aptly utilized form of light. Knowledge does not spread by keeping a lantern on one's own head but by spreading through the words and this book tries to be the ultimate source for the knowledge about lasers.

This book aims to be concise and precise guide to various laser applications in operative dentistry and endodontics. Laser light has made quantum leap into our routine dental practice ranging from cavity preparation to laser-assisted endodontics and cosmetics. Thus I have tried to introduce the lasers through a student's point of view and then further augmented the information by citing the studies done about the use of lasers in operative dentistry and endodontics.

Attempt has been made to include figures, tables and flowcharts for better and clear understanding of the subject. The journey of compiling the book has been truly humbling. I recommend it for all those who want to learn the use of lasers in dentistry, integrate their practice with lasers, and who consider it a new avenue.

I will be glad if the students, practising dentists, dental faculties and critics find it useful.

Vinisha Pandey

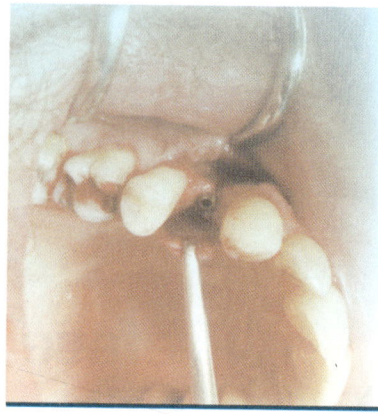

Acknowledgements

I bow in gratitude to the Almighty for giving me courage to venture out this work. Without His blessings, I could not have completed this book.

I would also like to thank Dr Donald Coluzzi, Health Science Clinical Professor, University of California, San Francisco School of Dentistry, whose invaluable suggestions was a driving force for my book.

I would like to extend my gratitude to Mr YN Arjuna of CBS Publishers & Distributors Pvt Ltd, New Delhi. Writing this book has been one of the most cherished aspirations and would not have been possible without the publishers' faith and encouragement.

Writing on various topics often requires a collective effort. I offer profound gratefulness and heartfelt thanks to my esteemed teachers Asheesh Sawhney and Abhinav Misra who have been very generous in extending their valuable help and suggestions at every step, whenever, I needed for this work. I am extremely thankful to them for their personal interest and dynamic enthusiasm which paved the way for smooth completion of my work. Their valuable suggestions and expert opinions have been a constant source of inspiration for me.

I would also like to sincerely thank Dr Vipul Srivastava and Dr Shally Mahajan of Association for Excellence in Clinical Dentistry (AECD), Lucknow, and Dr Bhuvan Jyoti (Dental Surgeon and Consultant in Oral Medicine and Radiology, Department of Dental Surgery, RINPAS, Ranchi, Jharkhand). They have been a major source of paving the path for this book.

Last, I am thankful to all those seen and unseen well wishers who have contributed to the completion of this work.

Vinisha Pandey

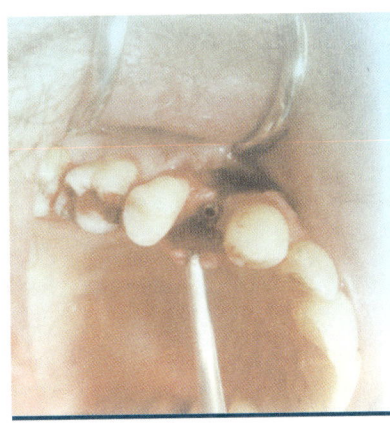

Contents

Foreword by Donald J. Coluzzi   *vii*

Preface   *ix*

1. *Introduction*   1

2. *Fundamentals of Laser*   7
   - Laser physics
   - Characteristics of laser light

3. *Technical Aspects of Laser Settings*   18
   - Stripping the fiber
   - Cleaving the fiber
   - Laser plume

4. *Laser–Tissue Interaction*   26
   - Condition for absorption
   - Effects of laser energy on oral tissues

5. *Classification of Lasers*   31
   - According to wavelength
   - According to physical construction
   - According to tissue on which it is used
   - According to potential hazards
   - Important laser types

6. *Lasers in Operative Dentistry*   40
   - Diagnostic laser application for detection of dental caries
   - Diagnostic laser application used as research tools
   - Lasers on hard tissue
   - Laser application in dental laboratory

7. *Low-Level Laser Therapy* — 80
   • Mechanism of LLLT
   • How does it work
   • Physiological changes
   • LLLT unit
   • Clinical applications in dentistry

8. *Lasers in Endodontics* — 89
   • Endodontic diagnosis
   • Pediatric endodontics
   • Laser-assisted endodontics
   • Fiberoptics and their modifications

9. *Esthetics and Lasers* — 115
   • Gingivectomy for tissue hyperplasia
   • Gingival cosmetic resculpturing
   • Frenectomy
   • Gingival troughing
   • Laser bleaching

10. *Laser Safety* — 122
    • Laser hazard classification
    • Non-beam laser hazards
    • Safety protocol
    • Laser safety officer (LSO)

11. *The Future of Lasers in Dentistry* — 129

12. *Before Purchasing a Dental Laser* — 134
    • Laser device checklist
    • International and national organizations dedicated to use of lasers

Glossary — 137

References — 144

Index — 151

1

Introduction

The word 'LASER' conjures in the mind's eye many aspects of what might be described as 'modern' life. The words 'powerful', 'precise' and 'innovative' complement our conception of the word in terms of technology whereas patients often associate the terms 'magical' and 'lightening quick' with the use of lasers.[1–3]

The word 'Laser' is an acronym for **light amplification by stimulated emission of radiation**. It is a technology that can amplify and produce a highly directional, intense, monochromatic and coherent beam.[99]

Laser is the mightier new *"avatar"* of light. The wonder beam has penetrated into normal life, more than any other form of concentrated energy.[99]

Today, laser is familiar to everyone because of its multifarious nature—be it in medicine, communication, industry/defense, etc. *almost anything and everything*.[99]

Lasers were first developed in the 1960s, and research into their applications in dentistry began soon thereafter. Early lasers were continuous wave devices with non- contact delivery that were found to be too hot for practical dental use. In the early 1980s, short-pulsed, fiber optic contact delivery laser technology was developed. Further technologic advances have led to smaller laser units, such as Nd:YAG and diode lasers.[74] In the past 15 years, dental lasers have had a huge growth in practical dental applications. Currently there are 20 specific indications, both soft tissue and hard tissue for use of a variety of dental lasers. However, no one device can accomplish all the practical dental uses. There has been continued growth in this new and maturing field of dentistry.[74]

Research is still ongoing in areas of caries prevention and areas of optical coherence tomography for undestructive imaging of enamel and dentin to determine lesion progression over time.[74]

HISTORICAL BACKGROUND OF LASER

1. Emergence of Laser Era

Laser is one of the most significant contributions of the last century to science.

The first successful demonstration of laser beam was done using ruby crystal by **Theodore Mainman** in the year 1960.[99]

With his contribution, we have lasers to help us progress in almost all scientific, technical, industrial, economic, social and medical fields.[99]

2. Lasers Today

The whole scenario changed and in came laser with a big–bang. Laser can be considered as a *successful offspring out of marriage between optics and electronics.* Laser action is usually demonstrated in different solids, gaseous substances, liquids, semiconductors, etc. ranging and radiating in thousands of wavelengths from millimeters to X-rays.[99]

3. Contribution of Albert Einstein

The theoretical basis that postulated the production of intense light of a specific configuration predated the development of first laser by over 40 years.[123]

In **1704, Newton** characterized light as stream of particles. The **Young's** experiment in **1803** and discovery of polarity of light convinced in the form of waves. The concept of *'Electromagnetic Radiation'* of which light is an example had been described in mathematical form by **Maxwell in 1880.** At the turn of 20th century, the 'Black Body Radiation' phenomenon challenged the waveform light theory. Atomic structure would absorb incident EM energy and become excited to an upper level which would significantly decay to lower stable state with the release of emissive energy.[123]

Additional work undertaken by **Hertz** on 'photoelectric effect' (a study on cathode ray emission) and **Planck** on the formulation of distribution of radiation emitted by black body or perfect absorber of radiant energy, complemented further understanding of light propagation. Planck showed that radiation, such as light, is emitted, transmitted and absorbed in discrete energy or quanta determined by frequency of radiation and value of Planck's constant.[123]

The observations that the electron released by the photoelectric effect is proportional to the intensity of light and frequency/wavelength determines the maximum kinetic energy of electrons.[123]

In 1905, **Albert Einstein** stated that light can be regarded as composed of discrete particles (photons), equivalent to energy quanta.[123]

Einstein assumed that a photon could penetrate matter where it would collide with an atom. Since, all atoms have electrons; an electron would be ejected from the atom by energy of photons with great velocity.[123]

In 1917, Einstein also predicted Zur Theorie der Strahlung (theory of wavelength) that when there is population inversion between upper and lower energy levels among the atom system it was possible to realize amplified stimulated radiation, i.e. laser light. Einstein called this process *stimulated emission of light, which is the back bone of laser.*[123]

4. Post-Second World War Experiments

During the period after World War II, scientists engaged in microwave spectroscopy in the USA started locking for a coherent radiation in the microwave region within the radio frequency level.[99]

In 1947, professor **Charles H Townes** at the University of Columbia, USA obtained a patent right to convert resonance of molecular absorption in the elements of circuits, such as, filters, frequency stabilizers, etc.[99]

5. Emergence of MASER

After professor Townes got the rights, he started working with microwaves and produced a device whereby this radiation could be amplified by passing it through NH_3 gas. This was the first **MASER (microwave amplification of stimulated emission of radiation)** which was development as an aid of communication systems and time-keeping (*'the atomic clock'*).[123]

However, it was realized that only a fraction of incident energy was converted into maser energy. [123]

By this time, optical engineers and enthusiastic student world have started clamoring for changing the name of this branch from MASER to LASER as light was the main source of action. So the name MASER vanished and the process of light amplification began to be known as LASER.[99]

In 1960, Theodore Mainman successfully demonstrated the operation of laser using a ruby crystal. Since then many scientists contributed in the development of different types of laser and till now lasers have reached many branches fulfilling ones needs.[99]

6. Important Landmarks in the Development of Lasers[96]

Year	Name of the Scientist	Achievement/Breakthrough
1916	**Albert Einstein**	Theory of light emission, concept of stimulated and spontaneous emission.
1952	**Charles H. Townes**	Discoverer/inventor of MASER (microwave amplification of stimulated emission of radiation) at Columbia University—awarded Nobel Prize in 1964.
1957	**Gordon Gould**	First document defining and coining the term LASER
1958	**Arthur L. Schwalow and Charles H. Townes**	First detailed paper describing' optical MASER credited with the invention of LASER

Year	Name of the Scientist	Achievement/Breakthrough
1959	**N.G. Basov**	Independently invented MASER at Lebedev Labs. and was awarded Nobel Prize in 1964. Also gave proposals for semiconductor lasers.
1960	**Theodore H. Mainman**	Invented first working laser based on ruby crystal on May 16th 1960 with a wavelength of 0.6943 micrometers.
1960	**Arthur L. Schwalow and Charles H. Townes**	Laser patented under number 2929922
1960	**Peter P. Sorokin and Merik J. Stevenson**	Second laser based on uranium development by IBM Labs (wavelength 2.5 mm)
1961	**Javan, Bennet and Harriot**	First gas laser, at a wavelength of 1.15 micrometers in a He–Ne gas mixture with neon as emitting atom
1961	**J.C. Polani**	Proposal of a chemical laser
1962	**Robert Hall**	Invention of semiconductor laser with a wavelength of 0.84 micrometers.

Year	Name of the Scientist	Achievement/Breakthrough
1962	**Fred Brech and Lloyd G. Cross**	First laser induced breakdown spectroscopy (LIBS)
1963	**C.K.N. Patel**	CO_2 laser with a wavelength of 10 μm.
1963	**N. Bsov**	Proposal for gas–dynamic lasers.
1964	**Geusic et al**	Stimulated emission of Nd:YAG laser.
1964	**Bob Thomas and H.M. Markos**	Demonstrated working of 1st Nd:YAG laser.
1964	**William bridges**	Argon–ion laser with a emission wavelength of 0.514 μm (xenon) and 0.488 μm (krypton).
1966	**Schafer et al**	Dye laser
1967	**Pimentel et al**	First hydrogen fluoride (HF) laser
1968	**M. Ross**	First pumped Nd:YAG laser
1969	**Tiffany et al**	First powerful CO_2 laser (kW range)
1970	**N.G. Basov**	First excimer lasers based on xenon (Xe^{2+})
1971	**John Madey et al**	Proposals for free electron lasers.
1978	**Walling et al**	Solid-state lasers based on Alexandrite.
1979	**Soda et al**	First surface emitting laser diodes.
1987	**D. Payne**	Development of Er:YAG laser
1999	**Kozuma et al**	First atom laser
2000	**Alferov and Kroemer**	Received Nobel Prize in the field of semiconductor physics for studying type of substances used to build semiconductor lasers.

7. Lasers in Dentistry

The theoretical basis of laser light production was developed some 90 years ago, the first laser was used on extracted tooth 47 years ago.[123]

It is perhaps some what surprising that commercially available lasers have been used in dental practice during the past 18 years. Associated with the launch of the 'first' dental laser, there was a level of type that quickly led to a combination of frustration for dentists and research that discredited or minimized many of the claims for clinical use.[123]

In dentistry, the use of laser is considered adjunctive in delivering a stage of tissue management conductive to achieving a completed hard or soft tissue procedure.[123]

Theodore H. Mainman had exposed an extracted tooth to his ruby laser in 1960.[24] However, in 1964, **Stern and Sogannes** began looking at the possible uses of ruby laser in dentistry. They began their laser studies on hard dental tissue by investigation the possible uses of ruby laser to reduce sub-surface demineralization.[24]

In 1965, **Goldman** was the first to irradiate the surface of tooth intraorally. He called this *"superficial oblation that was not painful to the patient."* He also studied the effects of pulsed laser on human caries.[1] The results of the study showed that effects varied from small 2 mm deep holes to complete disappearance of carious tissue with some whitening of surrounding sum of enamel, indicating extensive destruction of carious areas, along with crater formation and melting of dentine.[1]

CO_2 laser was the first laser to receive FDA clearance for oral use in 1976. The commercial availability of laser for dental applications began in 1989 under the name *'American Dental Laser'*.[123] This laser using an active medium of Nd:YAG emitted pulsed light and was developed and marketed by **Terry Myers, an American dentist.** Though low powered and due to its emission wavelength inappropriate for use on dental hard tissue, the availability of a dedicated laser for oral use

gained popularity among dentists. This laser was first sold in the UK in 1990.[123]

Other laser wavelengths using machines that were already in use in medicine and surgery and only slightly modified became available for dental use in early 1990s. Being predominantly argon, Nd:YAG, CO_2 semiconductor diodes, all these lasers failed to address a growing need amongst dentists and patients for a laser that would ablate dental hard tissue.[123]

In 1989, experimental work by **Keller and Hibst** using a pulsed Er:YAG (2,940 nm) laser, demonstrated its effectiveness in cutting enamel, dentin and bone. This laser became commercially available in the UK in 1995 and was shortly followed by a similar Er, Cr:YSGG (erbium, chromium: yttrium scandium gallium garnet) laser in 1997, amounted to laser armamentarium that would address the surgical needs of clinical dentistry in general practice.[123]

Essentially, the use of adjunctive surgical laser in dentistry has sought to address efficient cutting of dental hard tissue, hemostatic ablation of soft tissue and also sterilizing effect through bacterial elimination. Less powerful, non-surgical lasers have been shown to modify cellular activity and enhance biomechanical pathways associated with tissue healing, aid in caries detection and assists in curing of composites materials.[24]

The decision to include laser in everyday dental care will depend not only on financial consideration, as to how their use enhances practice profitability, the greatest factor in making that decision will be an understanding of now laser wavelength interact with oral tissue, together with an appreciation of now their use can improve patient management.[24]

2

Fundamentals of Laser

LASER PHYSICS

1. Meaning of "LASER"

The word LASER is an acronym for light amplification by stimulated emission of radiation. These words offer an understanding of basic principles of how a laser operates.[40]

Light: Light is a form of electromagnetic energy that behaves as a particle and wave. The basic unit of this energy is called *photon*.[40]

There are 3 measurements that can define the wave of photons produced by a laser. The first is *velocity* which is the speed of light. The second is *amplitude*, which is the total height of wave oscillation from the top of peak to the bottom on vertical axis. This is an indication of the amount of intensity in the wave: The larger the amplitude the greater the amount of useful work which can be performed. The third property is *wavelength*, which is the distance between any two corresponding points on wave on the horizontal axis. This is a measurement of physical size which is important in determining how the laser light is delivered to the surgical site and how it reacts with the tissue.[40]

Wavelength is measured in meters and the wavelengths used in dentistry are smaller units, such as microns (10^{-6} m) or nanometers (10^{-9} m). A property of waves that is related to wavelength is *frequency*, which is measurement of number of wave oscillations/seconds. Frequency is inversely proportional to wavelength; the shorter the wavelength the higher the frequency and vice versa.

Amplification: Amplification is a process which occurs inside the laser, with the help of various components (Fig. 2.1).

An *optical/laser cavity* is at the center of device. The core of the cavity is comprised of chemical elements, molecules or compounds and is called *active medium/gain medium*. Lasers are generically named for the material of active medium, which can be a container of gas, a crystal or a solid-state semiconductor.[40] There are 2 gaseous active medium lasers used in dentistry: Argon and CO_2, the rest that are available are solid-state semiconductor wafers made with multiple layers of metals, such as gallium, aluminum, indium and arsenic or solid rods of garnet crystal grown with various combinations of yttrium, aluminum, scandium and gallium and then doped with the elements of chromium, neodymium or erbium.[40] The active medium is positioned within the laser cavity, an internally polished tube with *mirrors,* one at each end of the optical cavity, placed parallel to each other and surrounded by external energizing input: *pumping mechanism/excitation mechanism,* either

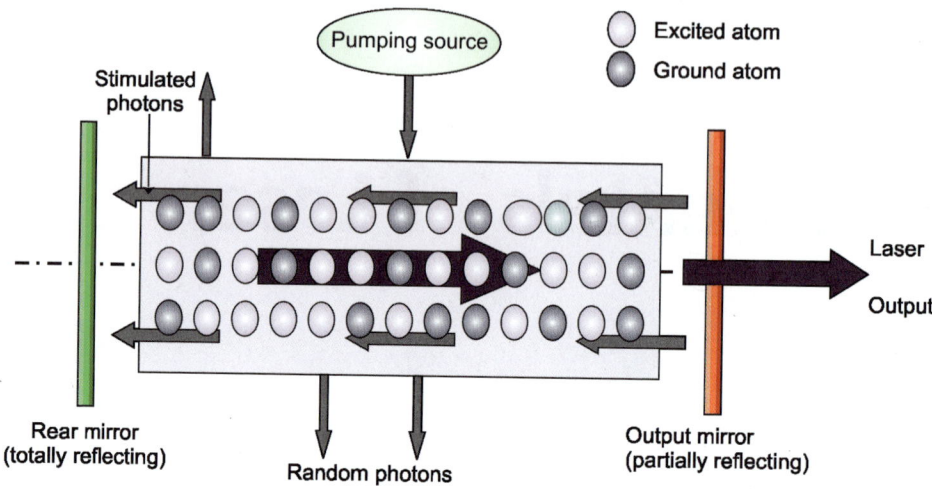

Fig. 2.1: Basic scheme of laser

a flash lamp strobe device or an electrical coil which provides the energy to the active medium. A *cooling system, focusing lens* completes the basic components.[40]

Optical resonator plays a very important role in the generation of laser, in producing high directionality to the laser and to overcome the losses due to straying away of photons from laser medium. This is achieved by bounding the laser medium between 2 mirrors. On end is high *reflectance mirror* (100% reflecting) or *rear mirror* and on other end are *partially reflecting/transmissive mirrors* also called *output coupler*. And it is this output coupler from which the laser bean emanates.[40]

Stimulated emission (Fig. 2.2): The term stimulated emission has its basis in the quantum theory of physics, introduced in 1900 by the German physicist *Max Planck* and further conceptualized to atomic architecture by *Niels Bohr,* a physicist from Denmark. A *quantum,* the smallest unit of energy, is absorbed by the electrons of an atom or molecule causing a brief excitation; then a quantum is released, a process called

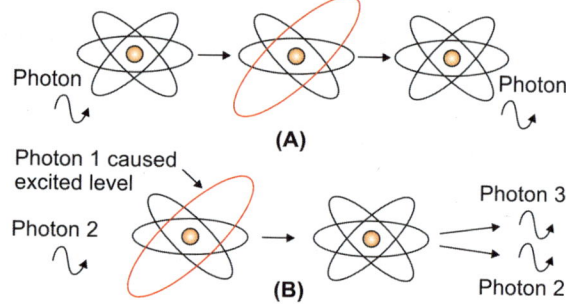

Fig. 2.2: (A) spontaneous emission (Bohr), (B) Stimulated emission (Einstein)

'*spontaneous emission*'. This quantum emission, also termed a photon, can be of various wavelengths because there are several electron orbits.[40]

Sir Albert Einstein proposed that an additional quantum of energy traveling in the field of excited atom that has the same excitation energy level would result in a release of 2 quanta, a phenomenon he termed as '*stimulated emission*'. This process occurs just before the atom could undergo spontaneous emission. The energy is emitted, radiated as 2 identical photons, traveling as a coherent wave.

The mirrors at each end of the active medium reflect these photons back and forth to allow further stimulated emission and successive passes increases the power of the photon beam. This is the process of amplification.[40]

Radiation: Radiation refers to the light waves produce by the laser as a specific from of electromagnetic energy. The electromagnetic spectrum is the entire collection of wave energy ranging from X-rays to radio waves whose wavelength can be thousands of meters. The very short wavelengths, those below approximately 300 nm are termed as *ionizing*. This term refers to the fact that higher frequency radiation has a large photon momentum, measured in electron volts/photon. Wavelengths larger than 300 nm have less photon energy and cause excitation and heating of tissues with which they interact. All dental laser devices have emission wavelengths of approximately 0.5 µm (or 500 nm) to 10.6 µm (or 10,600 nm). They are, therefore, within visible or invisible infrared non-ionizing portion of electromagnetic spectrum and exit thermal radiation. The dividing line between ionizing portion is the junction of ultraviolet and visible violet light.[40]

Electromagnetic Spectrum

The term 'Electromagnetic spectrum' refers to all forms of energy transmitted by means of waves traveling at the speed of light.[40] The electromagnetic spectrum extends from below frequencies used for modern radio (at long wavelength end) through gamma radiation (at short wavelength end) covering wavelength from thousands of kilometers of a fraction the size of an atom. Frequencies of 30 Hz and below can be produced and frequencies as high as 10^{27} Hz have also been detected.[123]

Higher frequency electromagnetic waves have a shorter wavelength and higher energy whereas low frequency waves have long wavelength and low energy.

Regions and Boundaries

Generally, electromagnetic radiation is classified by wavelength into infrared, ultraviolet and visible regions which is perceived by human being in the form of light.

Infrared Region

Infrared radiation is electromagnetic radiation whose wavelength is longer than that of visible light. The word infrared means *'below red'* being the color of visible light with the longest wavelength.[41]

It has a wavelength between 750 nm and 1 mm. Humans at normal body temperature can radiate wavelengths of 10 micrometers.[41]

Produced by molecular vibrations and rotations, i.e. heat and causes such motions in molecules of object that absorb it. Infrared band is divided into smaller section:
- *Far-infrared:* (25 to 40) to (250–300) µm
- *Mid-infrared:* 5 to (25–40) µm
- *Near-infrared:* (0.7–1) to 5 µm.

Visible Region

The visible spectrum also known as *optical spectrum* is the portion of electromagnetic spectrum that is visible to human eye electromagnetic radiation in this range of wavelength is termed as *visible light or simply light.*[41]

A typical human eye responds to a wavelength in the range of 380 to 750 nm.

The familiar colors of the rainbow in the spectrum include all these colors that can be produced by visible light of single wavelength only; the pure spectral monochromatic colors.[41]

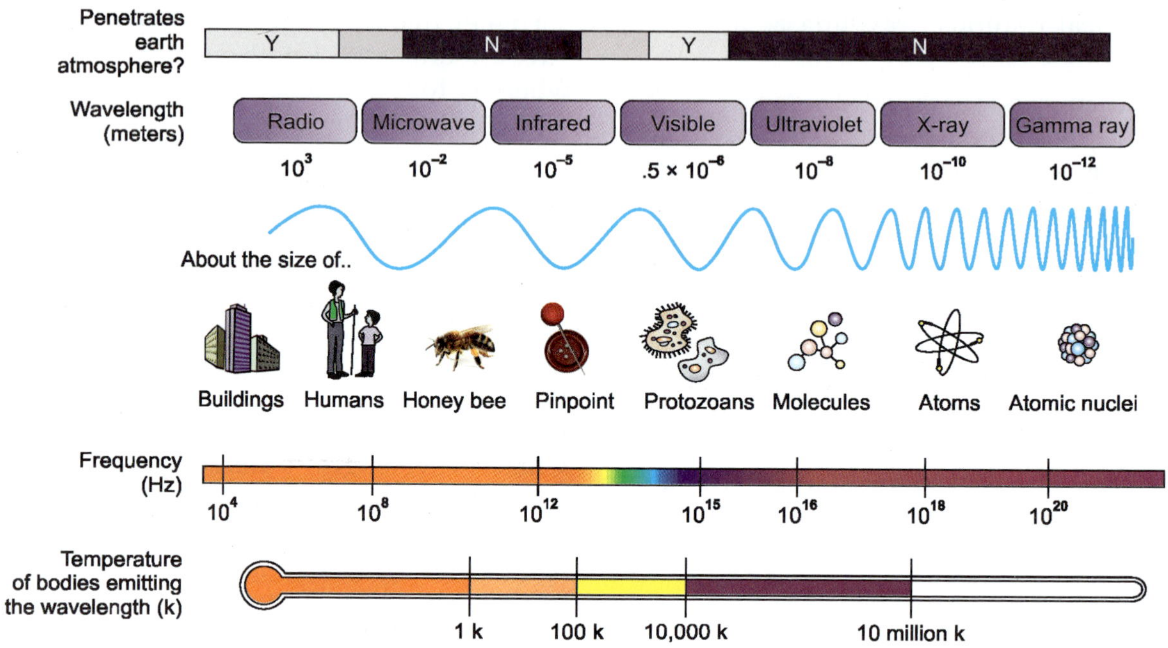

Penetrates earth atmosphere?					

Penetrates earth atmosphere? Y N Y N

Wavelength (meters)

Radio	Microwave	Infrared	Visible	Ultraviolet	X-ray	Gamma ray
10^3	10^{-2}	10^{-5}	$.5 \times 10^{-6}$	10^{-8}	10^{-10}	10^{-12}

About the size of..

Buildings Humans Honey bee Pinpoint Protozoans Molecules Atoms Atomic nuclei

Frequency (Hz)

10^4 10^8 10^{12} 10^{15} 10^{16} 10^{18} 10^{20}

Temperature of bodies emitting the wavelength (k)

1 k 100 k 10,000 k 10 million k

Fig. 2.3

Color	Wavelength (in nm)
Violet	380–450
Blue	450–495
Green	495–570
Yellow	570–590
Orange	590–620
Red	620–750

Ultraviolet Region

Ultraviolet radiation is electromagnetic radiation with a wavelength shorter than that of visible light, but longer than X-rays. It is named so because the spectrum consists of electromagnetic waves with frequencies higher than those humans identify as color "violet".[41]

The electromagnetic spectrum of UV light can be subdivided by a number of ways.

Name Wavelength (in nm) (Fig. 2.4)

	Wavelength (in nm)
1. Ultraviolet A (long wave)	400–315
Near	400–300
2. Ultraviolet B (medium wave)	315–280
Middle	300–200
3. Ultraviolet C (short wave)	280–100
Far	200–122
Extreme	121–10

The choice of an appropriate wavelength involves a combination of known tissue effect and operators clinical experience.

2. Laser Delivery Systems

Dependent upon emitted wavelength, the delivery system may be quartz fiberoptic flexible hollow wave guide, an articulated arm (incorporating mirrors) or a handpiece containing laser unit (for low-powered lasers).[123]

Articulated Arm

Before the introduction of Nd:YAG laser in 1990, most dental lasers used bulky articulated arm for their delivery system. It consists of a series of hollow tubes with mirrors at each

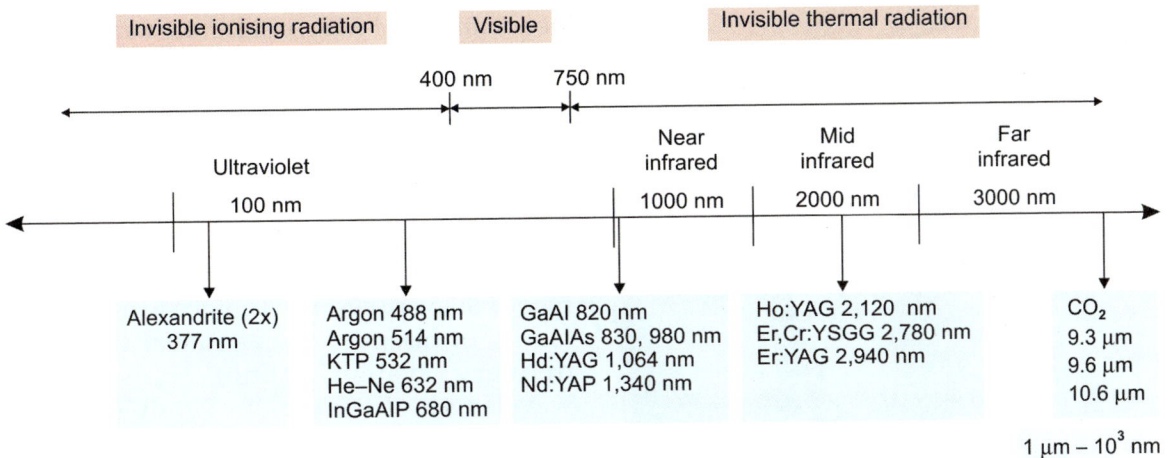

Fig. 2.4: Laser wavelengths commonly used in clinical dentistry[123]

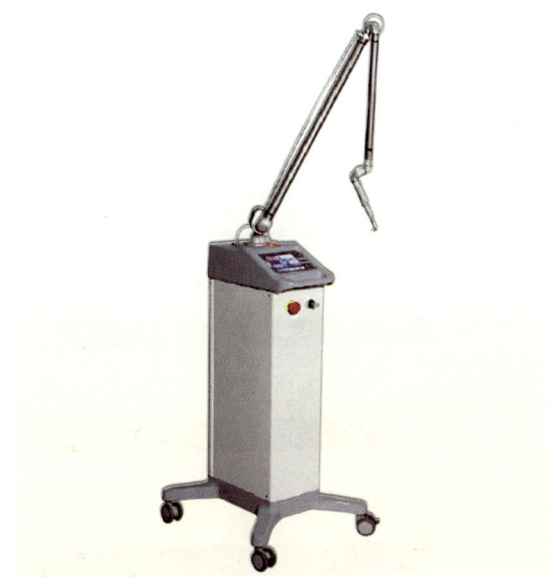

Fig. 2.5: Articulated arm delivery system. (*Courtesy: DEKA Laser Technologies LLC, Ft. Lauderdale, FL.*)

joint (called a *knuckle*) that reflect the energy down the length of tube (Fig. 2.5). This joint allows the delivery arm to be bent in such a way as to bring the handpiece close to the target tissue. The laser energy exits the tube through the handpiece. *Most commonly used with CO_2 laser.*[112]

Advantages

a. Tremendous flexibility of the arm allows rotation about the normal axis of mirrors.

b. Use of telescopic arms enables the length of arm to be changed.

Disadvantages

a. Awkward three-dimensional manueuverability of the arm which makes removal of discrete lesions difficult.

b. Bulky, difficult to use, non-contact mode, rigid, longer learning curve makes it not conductive for use in general dentistry.

Waveguide

Waveguide is a single, long semiflexible tube without knuckles or mirrors (Fig. 2.6). It consists of an inner reflective lumen along which the laser energy is transmitted and exits through a handpiece at the end of the tube which can be used either in contact or non-contact mode. Two types of waveguides which are used commonly with lasers: *Planar* and *Channel* waveguides. Planar waveguides guide light only in vertical dimension as in for laser-induced breakdown spectroscopy, whereas channel waveguides guide light in 2

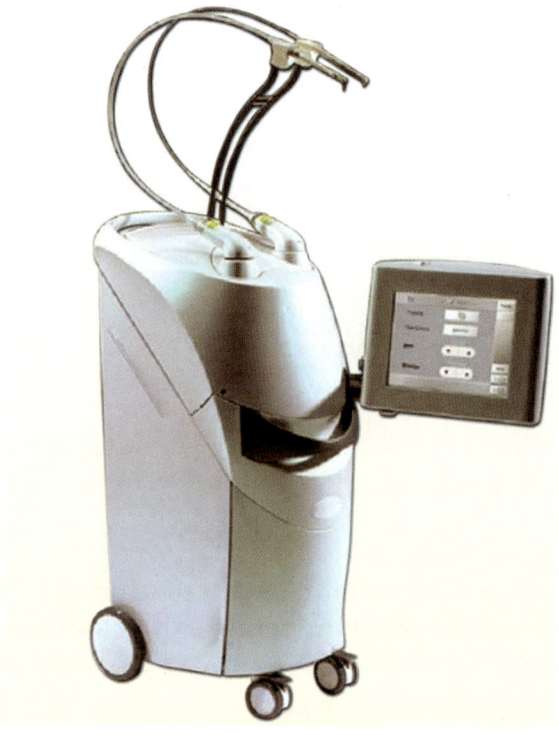

Fig. 2.6: Waveguide delivery system. (*Courtesy: Opus Dent, Santa Clara, CA.*)

dimensions. Used for conducting large wavelength lasers, like CO_2 lasers.[112]

Optical Fibers

The American Dental Laser dLase Nd:YAG system was the first such instrument to use a fiberoptic delivery system. This fiberoptic technology allows for contact with the target tissue (Fig. 2.7). The fiberoptic cables are attached to a small handpiece similar in size to a dental turbine and are available in sizes ranging from 200 µm in diameter to 1000 µm in diameter. Fiberoptic cables also are relatively flexible. This flexibility allows for easy transmission of the laser energy throughout the oral cavity, including into periodontal pockets. Laser light can be delivered by an optical fiber, which is frequently used with near infrared and visible lasers. Most commonly made of glass, i.e. silica. The light is trapped in the glass and propagates down through the fiber in a process called *total internal reflection.* Used for: Argon, diode, and Nd:YAG lasers.

The final delivery system is the **air-cooled fiberoptic delivery system** (Fig. 2.8).[112] This type of delivery system is unique to the erbium family of lasers. A conventional fiberoptic delivery system cannot transmit the wavelength of the erbium family of lasers, owing to the specific characteristics of the erbium wavelength. These special air-cooled fibers terminate in a handpiece with quartz or sapphire tips. These tips are used slightly (1–2 mm) out of contact with the target tissue.[112]

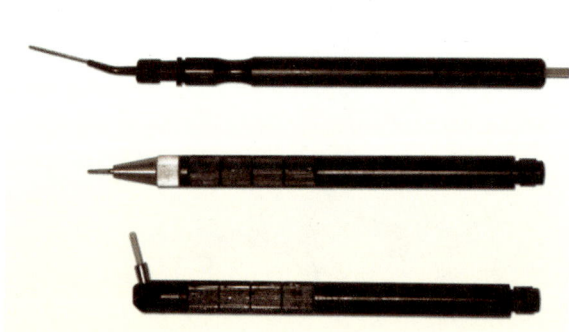

Fig. 2.7: Fiberoptic cables of various diameters and handpieces from a CO_2 waveguide delivery system

Advantages: Provide easy access and transmit high intensities of light with almost no loss.

Disadvantages: The beam is no longer collimated and coherent when emitted from the fiber which limits the focal spot size.

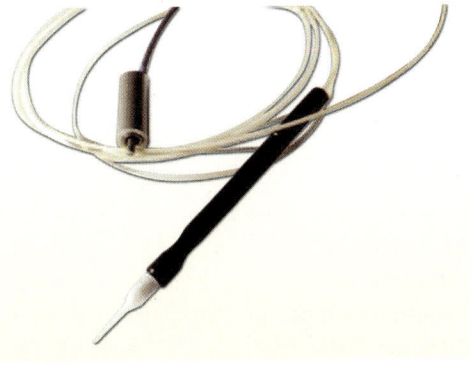

Quartz fiber

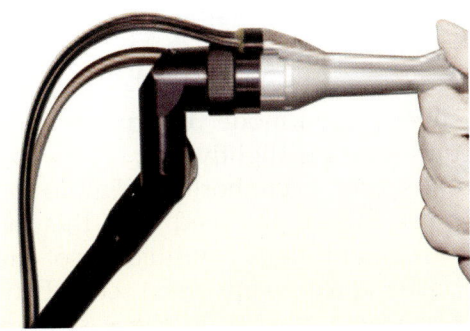

Articulated arm

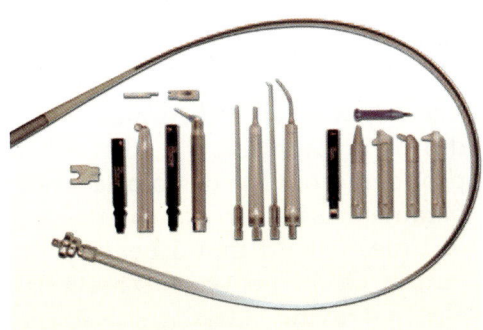

Hollow waveguides

Fig. 2.8: Types of laser delivery system

3. Emission Modes[123]

Once the laser is produced, its output power may be delivered in the following modes.

1. *Continuous wave:* When laser machine is set in a continuous wave mode the amplitude of the output beam is expressed in terms of watts. In this mode, the laser emits radiation continuously at a constant power levels of 10 to 100 W, e.g. CO_2 laser.

2. *Chopped:* The output of a continuous wave can be interrupted by a shutter that "chops" the beam into trains of short pulses. The speed of the shutter is 100 to 500 ms.

3. *Gated:* The term superpulsed is used to describe the output of a gated high peak power laser with short pulse duration, typically between hundreds of microseconds (1 ms = 1×10^{-6} sec). The pulse produced during superpulsing can have a repetition rate of 50 to 250 pulses per second that permits the laser output to appear almost continuous during use.

4. *Pulsed:* Lasers can be gated or pulsed electronically. This type of gating permits the duration of the pulses to be compressed producing a corresponding increase in peak power, that is much higher than in commonly available continuous wave mode.

5. *Super-pulsed:* The duration of pulse is one hundredth of microseconds.

6. *Ultra-pulsed:* This mode produces an output pulse of high peak power that is maintained for a longer time and delivers more energy in each pulse than in the super-pulsed mode. The duration of the ultra-pulse is slightly less.

7. *Q-switched:* Even shorter and more intense pulse can be obtained with this mode. Several hundreds of millijoules of energy can be squeezed into nano-second pulses.

8. *Flash-lamp pulsing:* In these systems, a flash-lamp is used to pump the lasing medium, usually for solid state lasers.

Laser types and their mode of emission are depicted in Table 2.1.

4. Laser Operating Parameters[(40)]

All the laser instruments used in dentistry feature parameters that are adjustable by the clinician; these are (Fig. 2.9):

1. *Energy* is the ability to perform work and is expressed as joules or millijoules. Energy = Force × Distance.

2. *Power* is the measurement of work completed over time and is measured in watts. { 1 watt = 1 joule/second }

3. *Average power* is the power that affects the tissue on a sustained basis over a period of time.

4. *Pulse duration/pulse width* is the total time that a beam is continuously producing

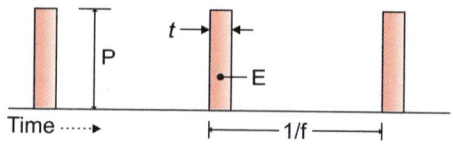

	Example
t Pulse duration (or pulse width) : 350 ms
P Pulse power = E/t : 2.29 KW
E Pulse energy : 0.8 J/pulse
f Frequency (or repetition rate) : 7 Pulse/s
P Average power = E × f : 5.6 W

Fig. 2.9: Anatomy of laser pulse

output. This time period determines the nature of 'true' pulsed laser versus gated system.

5. *Repetition rate:* The number of times during a given interval, that a beam is producing output on to a largest. This parameter is usually measured in number of time/second that a beam produces output. Cycles per second/hertz (Hz) are also synonyms.

6. *Power density* is the inherent power in the beam. Also known as **irradiance,** which is the amount of power/unit area. This parameter includes the nature of spot size, amplitude of wave and the specific wavelength involved.

$$\text{Irradiance} = \frac{\text{Power}}{\text{Area}}$$

Table 2.1: Laser types and their emission modes				
Type of laser	*Active medium*	*Wavelength (nm)*	*Mode of emission*	*Delivery system*
Gas lasers	Argon	488, 515	Continuous	Optical fiber
	Helium–Neon	633	Continuous	Optical fiber
	Carbon dioxide	9600, 10600	Continuous	Waveguide/articulated arm
Solid-state lasers	Nd:YAG	1064	Pulsed/continuous	Optical fiber
	Er:YAG	2940	Continuous/pulsed	Optical fiber/waveguide
	Er: Cr:YSGG	2780	Continuous/pulsed	Optical fiber
Semiconductor lasers	InGaAlP	655,810, 980	Continuous/pulsed	Optical fiber
	GaAlAs	830,980	Continuous/pulsed	Optical fiber
	GaAs	820	Continuous/pulsed	Optical fiber

7. *Energy density* is the sum total of fluent energy delivered to tissue from a direct source. It is also known as **fluence,** which is the irradiance multiplied by exposure time, measured in joules/square centimeter (Fig. 2.10).

Fluence or energy density determines the magnitude of laser interaction.

$$\text{Fluence} = \frac{\text{Pulse energy}}{\text{Area of spot size}}$$

The energy density (or fluence) determines the magnitude of the laser interaction

$$\text{Fluence} = \frac{\text{Pulse energy}}{\text{Area of spot size}}$$

• The spot size diameter (d) depends on the fiber core size (d_0) and the distance between the distal tip and the operating plane (h)

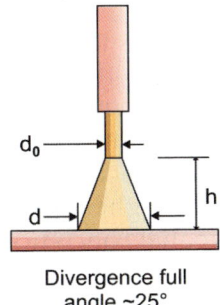

Divergence full angle ~25°

Fig. 2.10

8. *Beam diameter*: Lenses within the laser instrument focuses the beam. A beam of light incident on the tissue may be reflected, absorbed/scattered. Scattering in the tissue broadens the incident beam, decreasing the effective fluence in the intended target area. Doubling the spot size will increase the effective volume by a factor of eight. A large spot size usually enables faster and more effective treatment as in hemostasis.

As a general *rule*, doubling the spot size and having fluence will yield an effective fluence at a given depth. This effect becomes more pronounced with increasing depth.[40]

Mode of contact with tissues (relation of tip of delivery handpiece with tissue):[113]

1. Contact mode: Tip of handpiece in contact with target tissue.

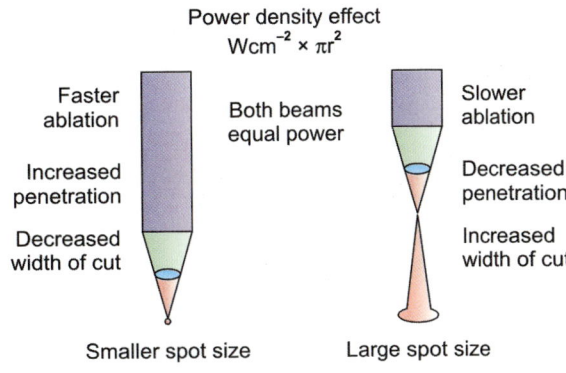

Power density effect
Wcm^{-2} × πr^2

Faster ablation

Increased penetration

Decreased width of cut

Smaller spot size

Both beams equal power

Slower ablation

Decreased penetration

Increased width of cut

Large spot size

Fig. 2.11

• Increased tactile sensation
• Increased access
• Focal point at or very near to the tip of delivery system.
• Used mainly with fiberoptic cable, for sharp incision or excisions.

2. Non-contact mode: Delivery tip at some distance from the target tissue.
• Decreased tactile sensation
• Access problem
• Focal point at some distance farther from tip.
• Used mainly with hollow waveguide for following tissue contours.

Beyond the focal point, the beam diverges and its power density and intensity decreases. When working on a tissue, the beam should always be used either with the focal point positioned at tissue surface (*focused*) or positioned above tissue surface (*defocused*). The lasers should never be positioned with focal point deep or within the tissue (*prefocused*) as it can lead to deep thermal damage and undesirable tissue effects (Fig. 2.12).

An important principle in any laser emission mode is that the light energy strikes the tissue for certain length of time, producing a thermal interaction. In the pulsed mode, the target tissue has the time to cool off before next

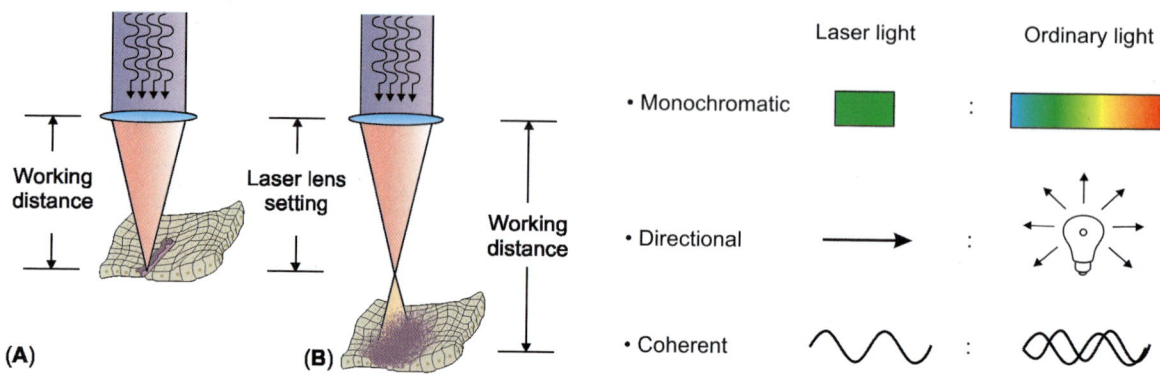

Fig. 2.12: (A) Laser-tissue interaction when the tissue is the focal distance away from the lens, Note the minimum beam diameter in the focal plane; (B) Laser-tissue interaction when the tissue is not in the focal plane of the lens. The laser covers a much larger area on the tissue surface

Fig. 2.13: Differences between ordinary light and laser light

pulse. But in continuous wave mode, operators must cease the laser emission manually to allow thermal relaxation.

CHARACTERISTICS (PROPERTIES) OF LASER LIGHT[109]

The significant feature of laser is the enormous difference between the character of its light and light from other sources, such as sun, a flame or an incandescent lamp (Fig. 2.13).

The most striking features of lasers are their:

1. Coherence
2. Monochromatic
3. Brightness and intensity
4. Directionality
5. Collimation
6. Focusability

1. Coherence

Laser light is said to be coherent which means wavelength of laser light are in phase of space and time, i.e. synchronized phase of light waves. Coherence can be spatial or temporal.

Spatial coherence: It is described as the phase relationship between waves traveling in a plane perpendicular to direction of propagation, i.e. waves travel side by side. Also known as *"transverse spatial coherence"*. For example, if we use a laser beam, the dark and light fringes falling on the screen will have the highest degree of contrast because of spatial coherence of laser.

Temporal coherence: It applies to waves traveling on the same path. Also known as *"longitudinal spatial coherence"*.

2. Monochromatic

Monochromatic refers to single wavelength (color) of laser beam. Ordinary white is a mixture of color as you can demonstrate by shining sunlight through a prism. Because the wavelength of laser light determines its effects on tissues; monochromatic property of laser light allows energy delivered to specific tissues in a specific way.

Thus, lasers are often defined by their visible color (e.g. red light/green light laser), by their position in the electromagnetic spectrum (e.g. infrared, ultraviolet or X-ray lasers) or by chemicals that create light (e.g. CO_2, argon and Nd:YAG lasers).

3. Brightness and Intensity

It is related to output power and beam quality of laser. All the properties of laser together produce a very intense and powerful flash or beam of light.

4. Directionality

Laser light is highly directional. It is emitted as a relatively narrow beam in a specific direction; whereas ordinary light is emitted in many directions away from the source.

5. Collimation

Collimation refers to parallel nature of laser beam. Laser light is emitted in a very thin beam with all light rays parallel to each other. All laser beams are parallel/collimated unlike regular light. Because the laser beam does not diverge significantly over distance, the source can be positioned at great length from target tissue or can be very efficiently focused down to a small spot with a convex focusing lens. Most solid-state lasers naturally emit collimated beams.

6. Focusability

Lasers work on the principle of stimulated emission of photons. These photons are released from their environment from first very small opening, because of the manner in which laser light is achieved it becomes highly focused, thus making lasers useful for specialized applications that require accuracy.

3

Technical Aspects of Laser Settings

When using a soft tissue laser both preparation of patient and preparation of laser are important. For this, well-trained staff should perform duties related to laser set up, patient explanation and preparation and clean up.

A sound knowledge of technical aspects of soft tissue laser is of paramount importance.

Prepare the Patient

The patient and the patient's guardian should be informed that most of the dental laser procedure will be performed under topical anesthetic and that most patients have no pain during or after the procedure. Past medical history should be recorded to allergies to anesthetic or any clotting abnormalities (e.g. hemophilia) or other medical contraindications to treatment. Discuss the advantages and disadvantages of the alternative procedures.

Informed consent should be obtained and the patient should be informed that results cannot be guaranteed and relapse may occur.

Once informed consent is obtained, isolate and dry the fields to assist with anesthesia. Apply topical anesthetic liberally over the site to be treated with laser.

An effective topical anesthetic for soft tissue procedures is TAC 20, a thin gel containing 20% lidocaine, 4% tetracaine, and 2% phenyl-ephrine with a shelf life of 3 months. However, topical anesthetic may be ineffective where isolation is difficult. In such situations, apply a topical anesthetic first and later injection anesthetic should be given for profound anesthesia. Gentle probing of the tissue should be done to confirm anesthesia. The patient should not feel anything sharp. The time required to reach anesthesia varies but in general start checking 3 minutes after placement of topical anesthetic.

Prepare the Laser

Arrange the laser unit next to the patient. Mostly all the units have a "key-lock" switch that should be turned "on" and a "ready/standby" switch which should be left on until the clinician starts the procedure. A prudent clinician should begin with minimal amount of power to accomplish the given procedure. Depending on the tissue thickness, for most tissue removal procedures, 1 to 1.4 W is a sufficient power setting; a higher power is rarely necessary.

Most diode lasers have two emission modes: Continuous wave (CW) and pulsed/chopped mode. A pulsed mode reduces the amount of heat to the surrounding tissues, but if the procedure can be carried out without charring continuous wave mode should be used.

Newer diode lasers have "superpulsed" mode in which laser emits very short pulses for a very short period of time. These lasers cut effectively with minimal charring than CW or gated pulsed mode.

The treatment objective, fiber size, and existing chromophore concentration should be considered when choosing the settings for a laser procedure.

FIBER

The fibers used with argon, diode, and Nd:YAG lasers are manufactured in a variety of diameters, with the 300 to 400 µ fiber most often used for laser procedures.

The fiber has 4 parts (Fig. 3.1): Coupler, cladding, jacket and fiber.

- The *jacket* is thick, flexible, clear or translucent, latex-like covering or a thin, tougher plastic that protects the fiber. Normally clear or white in color. When in operation, the jacket is stripped off on the working tip of the handpiece. A special tool is used for doing this.
- The *cladding* is a coating on the outside of the fiber that is inwardly reflective, collimating the laser beam completely to the fiber's terminal end.
- The *fiber* is itself made of quartz and is crystalline in structure.
- The *coupler* connects the fiber to the laser.

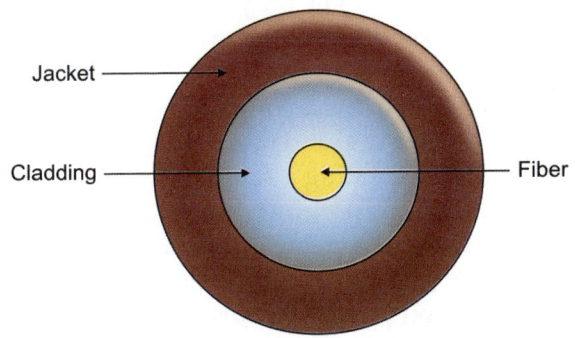

Fig. 3.1: Structure of an optical fiber

The fiber size can directly impact the amount of energy the target receives with a specific setting. A 320 µ fiber has a smaller spot size, which increases the power density at the target, compared with a 400 µ fiber. With the same setting, a 400 µ fiber delivers only 64% of the power density delivered with a 320 µ fiber.

Stripping the Fiber

When in operation, the jacket is stripped off on the working tip of the handpiece. A special tool is used for doing this. The jacket of a fiber is removed using a fiber stripping tool. When the laser outputs from the fiber tip, it is easy to retain debris from the tissues, the fiber tip is deteriorated. When the blackened tip extends 3–4 mm up the fiber shaft, it is time to cleave the fiber and strip the jacket to prepare a new tip for the next procedure.

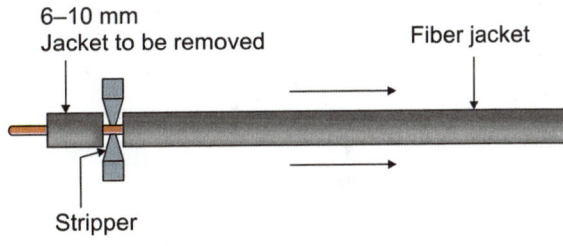

Fig. 3.2

Procedure

1. Insert the fiber end through the front hole of the stripper and grasp that portion of the fiber that will have the jacket removed between your thumb nail and index finger (Fig. 3.3).
2. Grasp the fiber with the stripper by applying pressure to the handles. With a slow steady force, remove the jacket of 6 to 10 mm by pulling the fiber away from the stripper (Fig. 3.4).
3. Pull the fiber out of stripper.

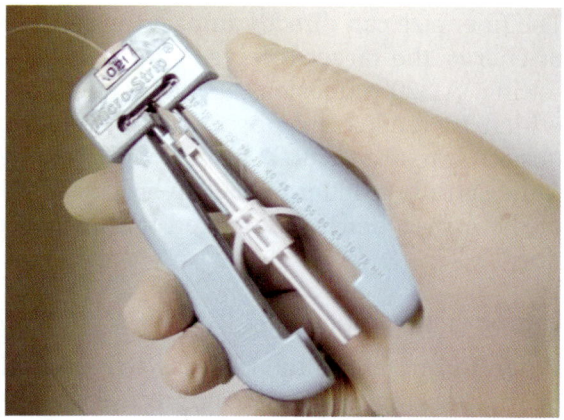

Fig. 3.3

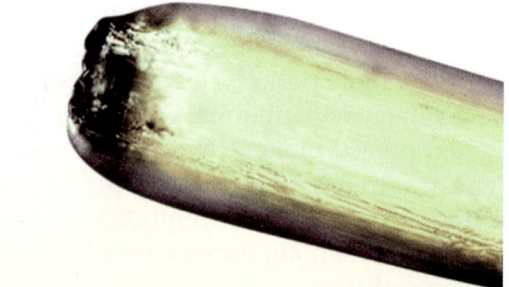

Fig. 3.5: Burned tip—needs cleaving

Cleaving removes the scratched part of the fiberoptic cable, exposing a fresh, highly polished cable surface capable of transmitting laser energy to the tissue.

Types of Cleaving Tools (Fig. 3.6)

- Carbide or diamond "pens" held at 90 degrees,
- 1 inch serrated ceramic tiles held at 45 degrees, and
- Scissors

Procedure (Fig. 3.7)

1. Lay the stripped fiber on a firm soft surface (a note pad works great for this and the glue strip on the back will hold the cleaved fiber for easy disposal.)
2. Put the cleaver blade gently on the fiber surface when you are ready to cleave.
3. Point the cleaver straight up and down and use a finger on your other hand to hold the fiber. You are now ready to cleave.
4. Push down on the cleaver not too hard (you need to try this a couple times to get the right pressure) and move the blade across the fiber creating a scratch in the fiber.
   Note: You are not trying to cut through the glass just create a flaw in the surface so the glass will break evenly.
5. After you scratch the surface, put the fiber between 2 fingers (be careful here) and

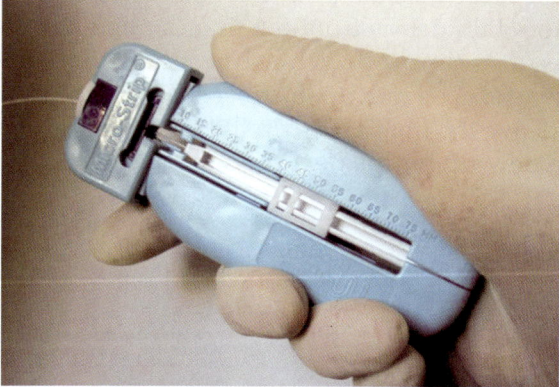

Fig. 3.4

Cleaving the Fiber

Cleaving refers to creating a flat, 90-degree surface at the terminal end of the fiber. This ensures maximum energy delivery from the fiberoptics.

As the tip deteriorates, it is more likely to fracture. To avoid this problem, it is prudent to periodically "cleave" the discolored tip (Fig. 3.5). It is standard protocol to cleave (cut) the fiberoptic cable at the end of each procedure to ensure laser is ready for the next procedure. After repeated use, fiber tip gets scratched and will not emit laser energy or ablate soft tissues efficiently.

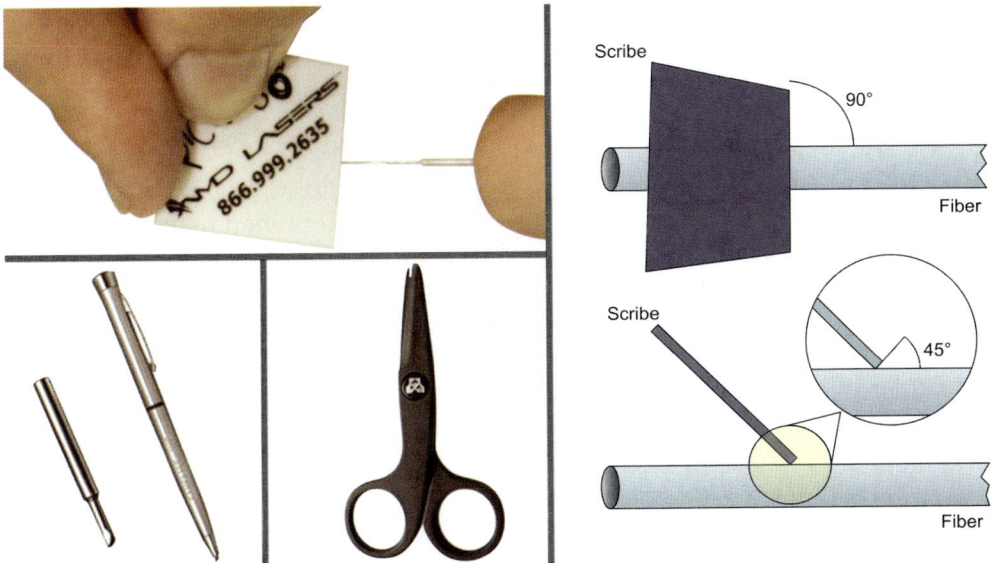

Fig. 3.6: Three types of cleaving tool: Glass cutting pen, scissors and ceramic tile

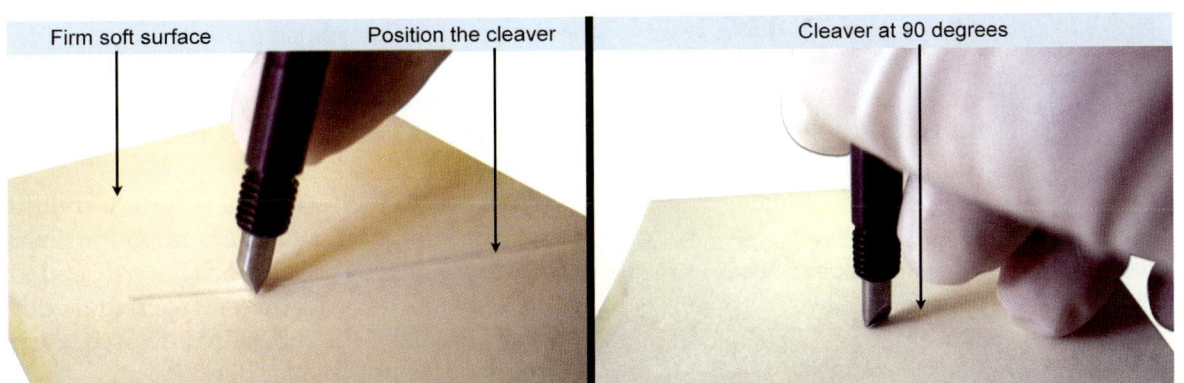

Fig. 3.7: Procedure of cleaving

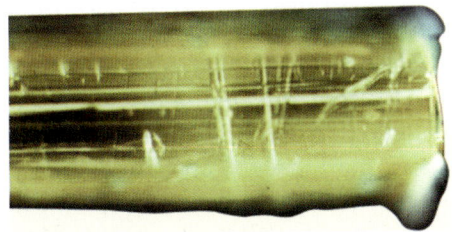

A well-cleaved fiber end

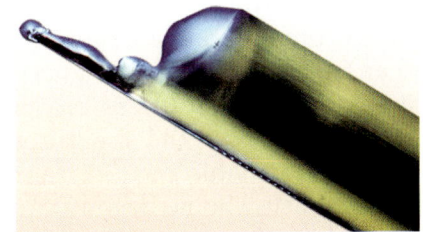

A poorly cleaved fiber

Fig. 3.8

pinch at the cleave point the fiber should break cleanly.

When glass cutting scissors are provided for cleaving, fiber is placed at 90 degrees between the blades allowing the fiber to scoot along the blade while closing them.

An optimal fiber cleave is checked by its aiming beam. The visible aiming beam should be a well-defined solid circle. A poor cleave creates an uneven or diffuse margin and may have a "comet tail" or oval appearance. An imperfect cleave diminishes the amount of laser energy being delivered to the target tissue and causes trauma when in contact with tissue. If the beam is irregular, re-cleave to obtain a clean cut (Fig. 3.9).

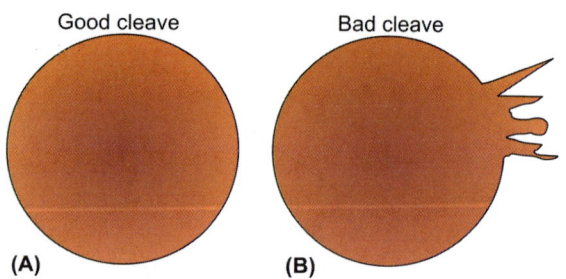

Fig. 3.9: (A) Appearance of aiming beam from a well-cleaved fiber; (B) Comet-tail appearance of unevenly cleaved fiber

A variety of handpieces are available for fiberoptic delivery systems. However, not every handpiece is compatible with every fiber. Fiber handpieces are available on the basis of body, barrel size, textures, etc. Most handpieces come with a chuck that tightens around an inner brushing. Due to crystalline nature of fiber, a cannula is required for guiding the fiber to the treatment site. Cannulas are available in metal and clear, transparent plastic. Some are multi-use and autoclavable, others are single use and disposable. Some may be shaped into an arc others may have a pre-defined shape (Fig. 3.10).

The clinician should consider these factors for an efficient, effective and comfortable working.

Using the Handpiece

- Care should be taken to avoid any damage to the jacket when using excessive turning force on the pressure nut. Only light pressure is required to secure the fiber firmly in place.
- Insert 15 cm of free end of the fiber through the pressure nut and the handpiece. Make sure that fiber end is stripped from insulation for about 2 cm on to the handpiece tip.
- Feed the end of the fiber through the disposable plastic tip/guide, while slightly twisting the tip and gently pushing the fiber through it. Firmly attach the tip.
- Most diode lasers use a plastic fiber guide. With the plastic guide, it is necessary to straighten the guide otherwise it can result in fracture or binding of fiber inside the guide.
- The lasers which use a metal guide should also be straightened while feeding the fiber. Once the fiberoptic cable has been extended to 3–4 mm beyond the end of metal tube carefully bend the tube to the desired angle taking care not to over bend it.

Initiating the Fiber

Some procedures call for the fiber tip to be 'initiated.' 'Initiation' prepares the tip of the fiber to retain heat by fusing a thin layer of pigment on the end. The process of initiating the tip will concentrate the laser energy in the tip essentially making it a "hot tip". The monochromatic laser light is turned into heat and hence this process is called photothermal reaction. The heat that is generated causes a localized zone of vaporization, surrounded by zones of carbonization (try to keep this char

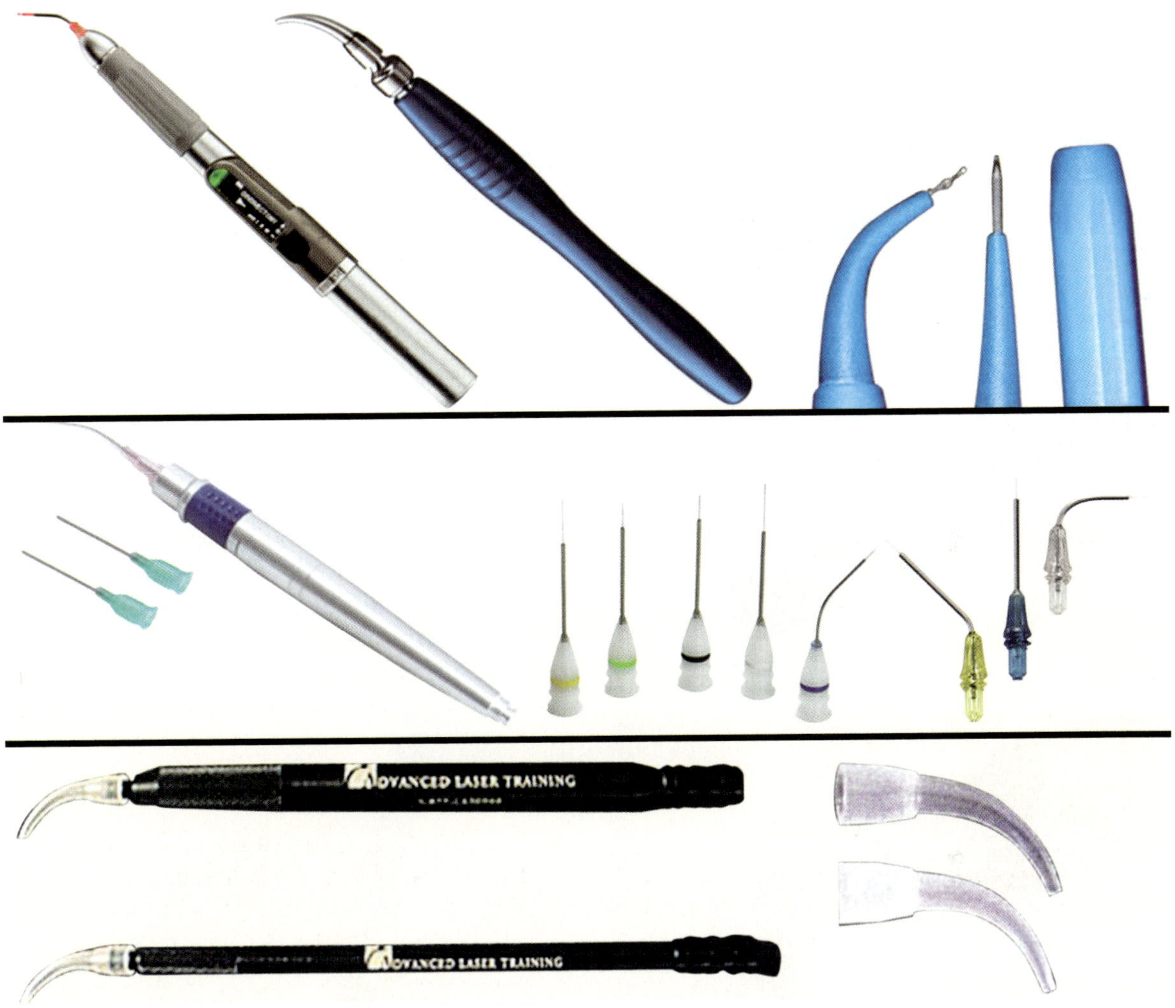

Fig. 3.10: Various handpieces and cannulas

zone as small as possible), coagulation and hyperthermia.

All soft-tissue lasers have a foot control option to activate the unit allowing a quick on or off when clinician is ready to ablate the tissue.

The easiest way to initiate a tip is by lightly moving the end of the fiber across a piece of articulating paper with the unit set to 1W CW. The tip will retain pigment from the paper and

will glow. Do not exceed contact time of 1–2 seconds.

If the objective is *penetration of the laser energy* into the tissue beyond the fiber, the fiber is *not* initiated. An uninitiated fiber is used for pre-procedural decontamination and coagulation. The Nd:YAG, a free-running pulsed laser, does not require initiating because of high peak powers and immediate interaction with the tissue. Argon and diode

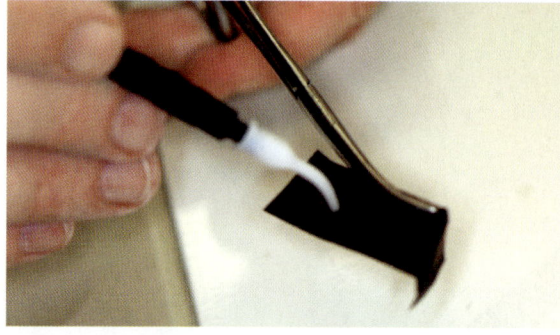

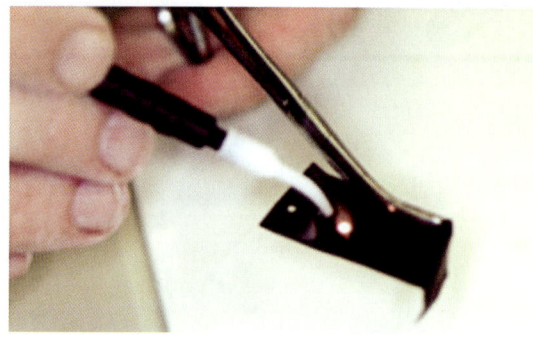

Tissue-laser interaction must be clearly understood for application of different temporal emission modes.

What purpose is served by the "Activation" of the diode dental laser tip?

The key to soft tissue removal with the diode laser is the carbon-rich black ink or char deposited on the diode laser fiber glass tip in order to "initiate" or "activate" it. The char absorbs the diode laser light and blocks it inside the glass tip. The glass tip then heats up to a temperature at which it can burn the soft tissue upon contact. Such thermal tissue removal is a slow heat-conduction process that depends on how charred and hot the glass tip is. Slow tissue removal induced thermal necrosis up to 6 mm deep is manifested by 1) extensive char left at the margins of incision, and by 2) white "seared" discoloration outside of the charred margins of incision (Fig. 3.11).

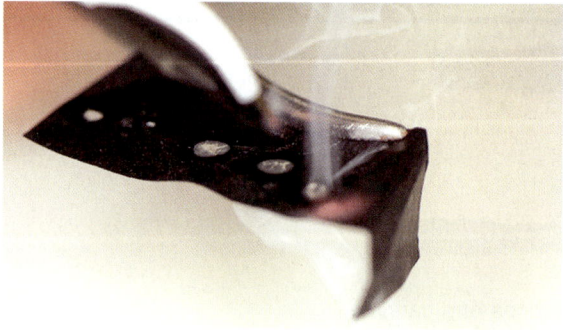

Fig. 3.11: Initiating the fiber using an articulating fiber

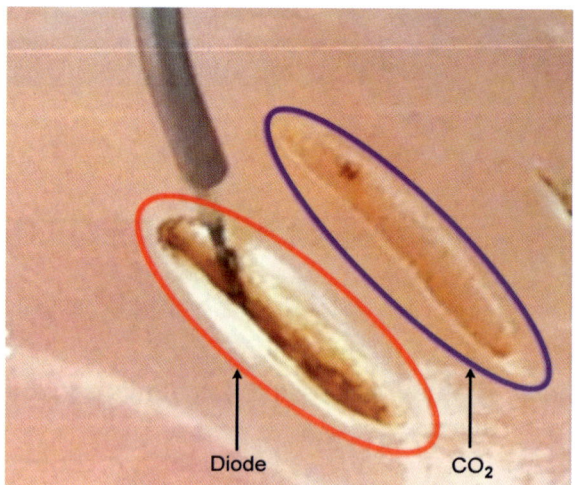

Diode CO_2

Fig. 3.12

lasers may be used in pulsed or continuous wave, with an uninitiated fiber for pre-procedural decontamination and coagulation. Continuous-wave mode requires less energy and shorter application time to minimize heat accumulation within the tissue. The pulsed-wave mode may use higher settings with slightly longer treatment times. The off time between pulses allows heat dissipation within the tissue.

Note

Test firing the laser before the patient's procedure is another important step in procedure preparation and safety. Test firing proves the laser energy is being delivered as

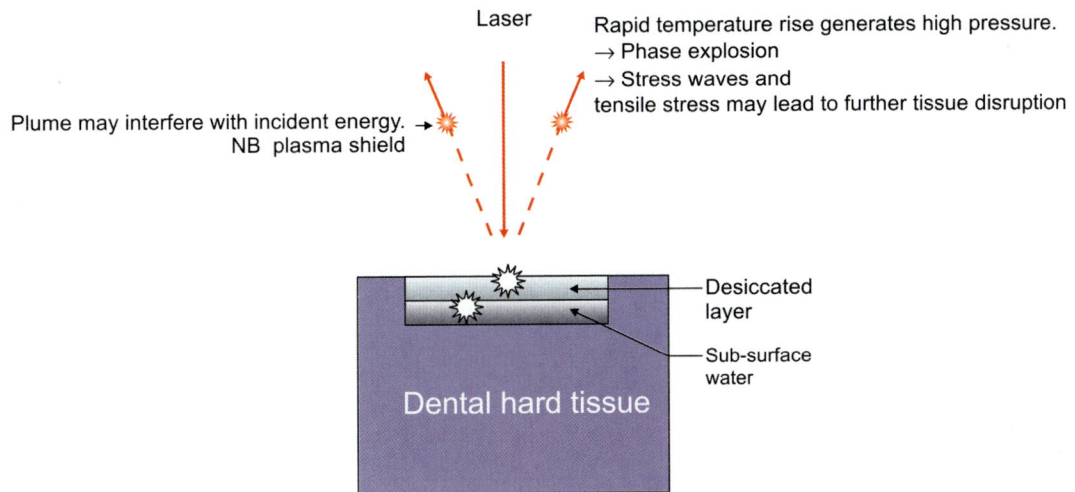

Fig. 3.13

expected. With safety measures in place, position the terminal end of the laser away from the patient. Select a suitable chromophore (argon, Nd:YAG, and diode: dark material; CO_2: moist paper; erbium: water) and activate the laser while holding it 1 to 2 mm from the material chosen. As energy is absorbed, an interaction will be observed, such as a mark and plume or water bubbling or evaporating. This is not the same as "initiating" the fiber, but simply an assessment to ensure the laser is working as anticipated.

Laser Plume

The plume is composed of 95% water and 5% particulate matter, organic and inorganic chemicals, and microorganisms. Organic chemicals, such as benzene, toluene, formaldehyde, and cyanide, have also been found (Fig. 3.13). Inorganic chemicals include carbon monoxide, sulfur, and nitrogen compounds. The microorganisms found were bacteria, microbacteria, fungi, viruses, and DNA from intact viruses of human immunodeficiency virus (HIV), hepatitis B virus (HBV), and human papillomavirus (HPV). Most particles are 0.3 to 0.5 μ in size. A mask filtering 0.1 μ particles is recommended. 0.1 micron filtration masks are available in tie or ear-loop style or tuberculosis style. High speed evacuation methods also assist in reducing and collecting the plume during lasing.

4
Laser–Tissue Interaction

When electronic energy (incident radiation) interacts with tissue, the tissue reflects part, the tissue absorbs part, and the tissue transmits and scatters part of the light. The surgical interaction of this radiant energy with tissue is caused only by that portion of the light that is absorbed, that is the incident radiation minus the sum of the reflected and transmitted portions (Polanyi, 1983).[24]

Laser light can have four different interactions with the target tissue depending on the optical properties of that tissue. Dental structures have complex composition and these four phenomenona occur together in some degree relative to each other.[40]

The first and the most desired interaction is the **absorption** of the laser energy by the intended tissue. The amount of energy that is absorbed by the tissue depends on tissue characteristics, such as pigmentation and water content and on the laser wavelength and emission mode.[40]

The main absorbing components or chromophores (tissue compounds) of tissue are:
1. Water (present in all the biologic tissues)
2. Hemoglobin in blood
3. Melanin of skin, hair
4. Protein and other macromolecules

Hemoglobin, the molecule that transports oxygen to tissue, reflects red wavelength imparting color to the arterial blood. It is, therefore, absorbed by blue and green wavelengths.[40] Venous blood, containing less oxygen, absorbs more red light and appears darker. The pigment melanin, which imparts color to the skin, is strongly absorbed by short wavelengths. Water, the universally present molecule, has varying degree of absorption by different wavelengths.[40]

Condition for Absorption

Dental structures have different amounts of water content by weight. A ranking from lowest to highest would show enamel (with 2–3%), dentin, bone calculus, caries and soft tissue (at about 70%).[40] Hydroxyapatite is the chief crystalline component of dental hard tissues and has a wide range of absorption depending on the wavelength.[40]

In general, shorter wavelengths (500–1000 nm) are readily absorbed in pigmented tissue and blood elements. Argon is highly attenuated by hemoglobin.[40] Diode and Nd:YAG has a high affinity for melanin and less interaction with hemoglobin (Fig. 4.1). The longer wavelengths are more interactive with water and hydroxyapatite. The largest absorption peak for water is just below 3000 nm which is at Er:YAG wavelength. Erbium is also well absorbed by hydroxyapatite. CO_2

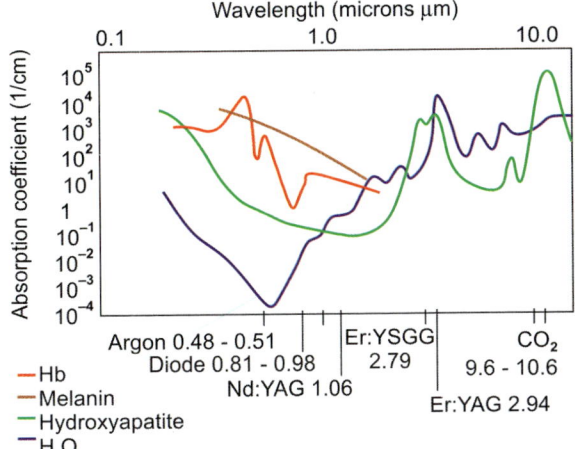

Fig. 4.1: Approximate absorption curves of the prime oral chromophores

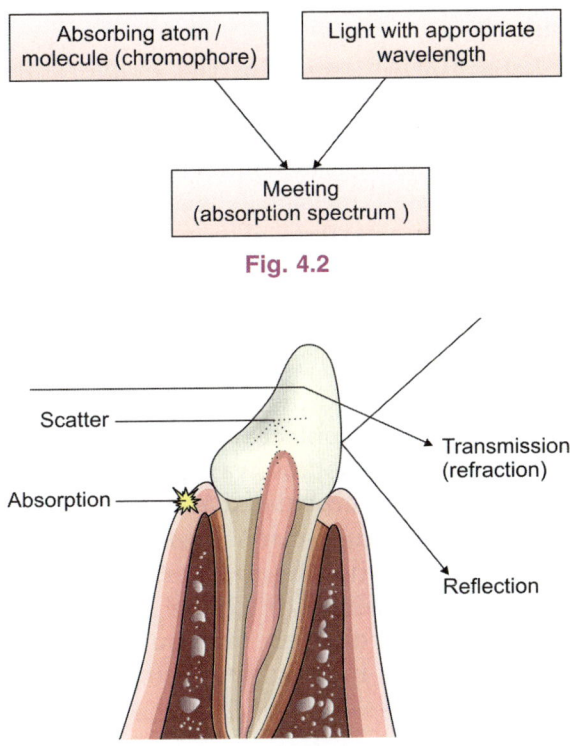

Fig. 4.2

Fig. 4.3

at 10,600 nm is well absorbed by water and has greatest affinity for tooth structure.[40]

The second effect is **transmission** of the laser energy directly through the tissue with no effect on target tissue, i.e. inverse of absorption. This effect is highly dependent on wavelength of laser light. Water, for example, is relatively transparent to the shorter wavelengths, like argon, diode and Nd:YAG, whereas tissue fluids readily absorb the erbium family and CO_2 at the outer surface so that there is little energy transmitted to adjacent tissues.[40]

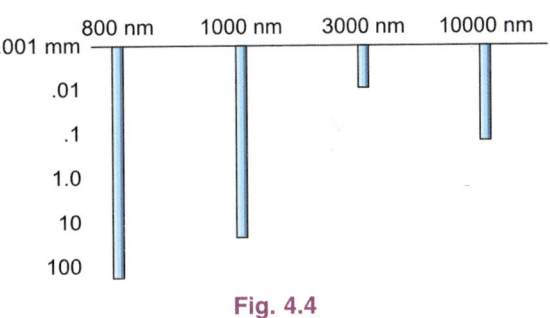

Fig. 4.4

Figure 4.4 shows this interaction by showing relative depth of penetration in water of various wavelengths. The depth of the focused laser beam varies with the speed of movement and the power density. In general, erbium family acts mainly on the surface, with an absorption depth of approximately 0.01 mm, whereas the 800 nm diodes are transmitted to the tissue to depths of up to 100 mm, a factor of 10,000. As another example, diode and Nd:YAG laser are transmitted through the lens, iris and cornea of eye and absorbed on the retina.[40]

The third effect is **reflection**, which is the beam redirecting itself off the surface having no effect on the target tissue. Caries-detecting laser device uses the reflected light to measure the degree of sound tooth structure. The reflected light could maintain its collimation in a narrow beam or become more diffuse. The laser beam generally becomes more divergent as the distance from the handpiece increases. However, the beam from some lasers can have adequate energy at distances over 3 m. This reflection can be dangerous because the energy is directed to an unintentional target, such as the eyes.[40]

The fourth effect is **scattering** of laser light, weakening the intended energy and possibly producing no useful biologic effect. Scattering of laser beam could cause heat transfer to the tissues adjacent to the surgical site and unwanted damage could occur (Fig. 4.5).[40]

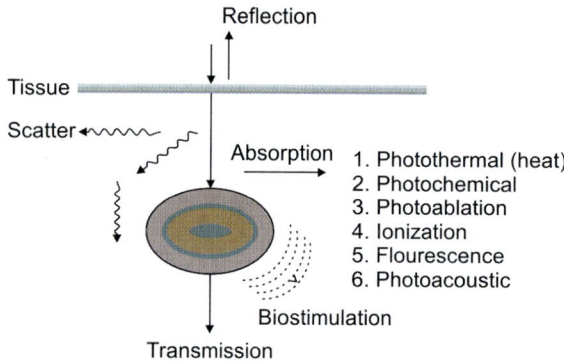

Fig. 4.5: Effects of laser–tissue interaction

Effects of Laser Energy on Oral Tissues

Absorption of laser light by the target produces effects which are beneficial and primary of laser energy.

The principal effect of laser energy is *photothermal* (i.e. conversion of light energy into heat). This thermal effect of laser energy on tissue depends on the degree of temperature rise and the corresponding reaction of interstitial and intercellular water. The rate of temperature rise plays an important role in this effect and is dependent on several factors, such as cooling of surgical site and the surrounding tissue's ability to dissipate the heat. As the laser energy is absorbed, heating occurs (Table 4.1).[40]

Table 4.1: *Laser energy and thermal effects on dental soft tissue*

Tissue temperature (°C)	Observed effect
37–50	Hyperthermia
60–70	Coagulation, protein denaturation
70–80	Welding
100–150	Vaporization, ablation
> 200	Carbonization

Hyperthermia occurs when the tissue is elevated above normal temperature but is not destroyed. At temperatures of approximately 60°C, proteins begin to denature without any vaporization of underlying tissue. The tissue whitens or blanches which is useful in surgical cases.[40]

Coagulation refers to the irreversible damage to tissue, congealing liquid into a soft semi-solid mass. This produces the desirable effect of hemostasis by contraction of the wall of the vessel.[40] Incision is accomplished by placing the laser at its focal length (i.e. smallest possible spot size) near the tissue or touching the tissue, if a contact tip is used. This increases the density of the power and condenses the effect into a small area. This laser target distance varies according to delivery system and ranges from contact with a contact laser to 0.5 mm for a hollow waveguide to more than 1 cm for an articulated arm laser.[76]

Soft tissues' edges can be **welded** together with a uniform heating to 70 to 80°C where there is adherence of layers because of stickiness to collagen molecules helical unfolding and intertwining with adjacent segments.[43]

When the target tissue containing water is elevated to a temperature of 100°C, **vaporization** of water occurs, also known as **ablation**.[43] This allows removal of large areas of very superficial epithelium the laser away from the target, to increase the spot size.[73] Defocusing effectively lowers the density of the laser energy/units and causes the laser to act more superficially over a larger surface area. The target distance may vary dramatically depending on the type of delivery system, the available power and the desired depth of penetration.[76]

The apatite crystals and other minerals in dental hard tissue are not ablated at this temperature, but the water component is vaporized and the resulting jet of steam expands and then explodes the surrounding matter into small particles. This mixture of steam and solids is then suctioned away. This micro-explosion of apatite crystal is termed **"spallation"**.[40]

If the tissue temperature continues to be raised to about 200°C, it is dehydrated and then burned in the presence of air, carbon, as the end-product, absorbs all wavelengths. Thus, if laser energy continues to be applied, the surface carbonized layers absorb the incident beam, becoming a heat sink and preventing normal tissue ablation (Fig. 4.6).[40]

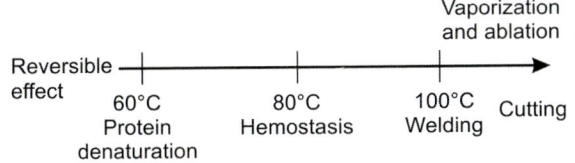

Fig. 4.6: A graphic representation of effects of laser light on dental tissues

Thus for dental applications, excessive heat must be avoided to protect the pulp.

THERMAL EFFECTS

Photochemical effects cause target cells to start light-induced chemical reactions (e.g. curing of composite resins) and breaking of chemical bonds (e.g. using photosensitized

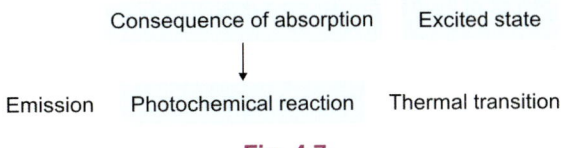

Fig. 4.7

drugs exposed to laser light to destroy tumor cells, a process called *photodynamic therapy*). Initial absorption takes place by specific molecules.[76]

Some of the applications of photochemical effects are:

1. Photo-activated dye disinfection using lasers
2. Photo polymerization of light-cured restorative resin using argon laser.
3. Photochemical bleaching

A laser can be used with powers well below the surgical threshold for **biostimulation (low-level laser therapy)** producing more rapid wound healing, pain relief, increased collagen growth and a generalized anti-inflammatory effect.[40]

For very high rates of energy deposition, shock waves can be generated in the tissue by mechanisms, such as bubble expansion/plasma formation. It causes dielectric breakdown in tissue caused by shock wave plasma expansion resulting in localized mechanical rupture.[76]

The pulse of laser energy into a crystalline structure can produce an audible shock wave, which could explode or pulverize the tissue with mechanical energy. This is an example of **photo-acoustic effect** of laser light.[40]

To Summarize

Effects of laser light on tissues
- Reflection
- Scattering/dispersion
- Absorption
- Transmission

Effects of light energy on target tissues
- Photothermal effects
  - Coagulation
  - Vaporization
- Photo-acoustic effect
  - Disruption
  - Plasma effect
- Flourescence
  - Caries detection
  - Mucosal evaluation
  - Photochemical effects
  - Stimulate chemical reaction
  - Breaks and creates chemical bonds
- Photo-biomodulation
  - Pain relief
  - Wound healing

Variables affecting laser–tissue interaction
- Wavelength
- Target composition
  - Chromophore—substance that absorbs light energy
  - Fluorophores—substances that emit/ produce light often when stimulated with light energy
- Interaction time
  - Temporal modes—continuous, pulsed or gated
  - Hand speed
  - Total interaction time
- Power
- Energy transfer mode—contact vs non-contact
- Spot size: Fiber size (320 μ vs 200 μ diameter)
- Operators knowledge and experience

Tissue interaction is maximized by matching the proper wavelength with adequate amount of power with the chromophore present in the tissue.

5

Classification of Lasers

Traditionally, lasers have been classified according to:

- The wavelength.
- The physical construction of the laser (e.g. gas, solid-state, liquid or semiconductor diode) and the type of medium which undergoes lasing (e.g. erbium: yttrium aluminum garnet, etc.).
- Tissues on which it is used: Soft and hard tissues.
- The degree of hazard to the skin or eyes following inadvertent exposure.

A. According to Wavelength[74]

1. *Ultraviolet/excimer laser*: The wavelength ranges approximately from 150 to 350 nm. The term 'excimer' is derived from two terms "excited dimer" which is an elevated energy state known for rapid dissociation into small particles of energy. Excimer laser exhibits high peak power level, at approximately 10–15 Hz and produces remarkably clean cuts in tissue. However, it has a great potential for causing mutagencity and cytotoxicity in various types of soft tissue (Arcoria, 2006).

2. *Visible light laser:* The visible light range is between 350 and 750 nm. The first laser of this category was ***ruby laser*** (633 nm) which was also the first laser to be constructed. ***Argon lasers*** (λ = 488.5 nm ***blue***; λ = 514.5 nm ***green***) lie in the middle of visible portion of the electromagnetic spectrum. Argon lasers are absorbed well in the red pigmentation especially blood and have a pronounced coagulative/hemostatic effect without affecting bone or tooth structure. Dye is most readily absorbed by blue pigmentation. ***Helium–neon*** (λ = 632 nm) is one of the more common types of low-powered (0.5 W) visible light laser used for low level laser therapy (Arcoria, 2005).

3. *Infrared laser*: This class of laser encompasses the most common type that is readily available in the market place. The wavelength range is between 730 nm and 12,000 nm. ***Nd:YAG*** (Neodymium: yttrium aluminum garnet; λ = 1064 nm) lasers are one of the most popular among these lasers. The wavelength is readily absorbed into black pigmentation and has a high degree of penetration into light-colored tissue using continuous wave (CW) mode.

   Ho:YAG (Holmium: yttrium aluminum garnet; λ = 2100 nm) lasers are used commonly for minimal cutting of tooth structure or recontouring of bone.

   Er:YAG (Erbium: yttrium aluminum

garnet; $\lambda = 2900$ nm) laser is one of the newer and promising type of 'hard tissue" laser. **CO$_2$** (Carbon dioxide; $\lambda = 9300, 9600, 10300, 10,600$ nm) laser is one of the oldest dental lasers. The wavelength is readily absorbed into water and hydroxyapatite and follows a surface-cutting mechanism.

4. *Tunable lasers*: These lasers can access a wide variety of wavelengths.

B. According to the Physical Construction and Type of Lasing Medium[99]

Table 5.1 describes the classification of laser according to physical construction and type of lasing medium.

Table 5.1: Classification of laser according to physical properties and lasing medium

Active medium	Physical construction	Wavelength (in nm)
1 Argon	Gas laser	488,515 nm
2 He–Ne	Gas laser	633 nm
3 Nd:YAG	Solid-state	1064 nm
4 Er:YAG	Solid-state	2940 nm
5 Er, Cr: YSGG	Solid-state	2780 nm
6 CO$_2$	Gas laser	9600 nm, 10300 and 10600 nm
7 Diode	Semiconductor laser	635–980 nm

C. According to the Tissue on which it is Used[128]

1. **Soft tissue lasers** (used for incision, excision and ablation) serve as a useful addition to soft tissue therapies and enable the dentist to treat the patient with extreme accuracy. The light vaporizes matter, delivering a narrow beam and promising precision. Soft tissue lasers are used for intraoral biopsy treatments. These treatments include removal of fibromas, wounds and oral papillomas. Soft tissue can also be used to shave gum tissue and to help root planning.

2. **Hard tissue lasers** (act by coagulation, vaporization, re-crystallization, charring and carbonization) are predominantly used for caries removal, cavity preparation and laser etching. Hard tissue lasers are used to treat minor or average sized cavities, bone surgery, bone incision, bone shaping and crown lengthening. Combined with water spray and laser energy, water containing tissue, such as the tooth structure, absorbs that energy.

D. According to Potential Hazards[40]

Class I : Fully enclosed system.

e.g. Nd:YAG laser welding system used in a dental laboratory, laser printers.

Class II : Visible low power lasers protected by blink reflex

e.g. Visible red aiming beam of a surgical laser, bar code scanners

Class IIIa : Visible lasers above 1 milliwatt. Have a caution label on them.

e.g. No dental example.

Class IIIb : Higher power laser unit (up to 0.5 watts), which may or may not be visible. Direct viewing hazardous to eyes.

e.g. Low power (50 milliwatt) diode laser used for biostimulation, argon curing laser.

Class IV : Damage to eye and skin possible. Direct or indirect viewing hazardous to eyes.

e.g. All lasers used for oral surgery, whitening and cavity preparation.

IMPORTANT LASER TYPES USED IN OPERATIVE AND ENDODONTICS

1. *Neodymium:* Yttrium Aluminum Garnet (Nd:YAG) Laser

Nd:YAG (Neodymium-doped yttrium aluminum garnet; Nd: $Y_3 Al_5 O_{12}$) is a crystal that is used as a lasing medium for solid-state laser. The dopant, triply ionized neodymium, typically replaces yttrium in the crystal structure of yttrium aluminum garnet since they are of similar size. Generally, the crystalline host is doped with around 1% neodymium. Laser operation of Nd:YAG was first demonstrated by *Geusic* et al at Bell Labs in 1964.[99] The active medium is different from gas or diode lasers and pumping mechanism is via a flash lamp. It has an emission wavelength of 1064 nm which is in the near infrared portion of electromagnetic spectrum.

It operates in a free running pulse mode with short pulse duration in hundreds of micro-seconds and features small flexible bare optical fibers that can contact the tissue.[99] The laser energy is highly absorbed by melanin but is less absorbed by hemoglobin, 90% of which is transmitted through water.

Nd:YAG optical fiber needs to be cleaved and cleaned; otherwise laser light will rapidly loose its effectiveness. When used in non-contact defocused mode, this wavelength can penetrate several millimeters, which can be used for produces, such as homeostasis treatment of aphthous ulcers or pulpal analgesia.[99]

Applications

1. Gingival troughing.
2. Esthetic contouring of gingiva.
3. Treatment of oral ulcers.
4. Frenectomy and gingivectomy.
5. Removal of incipient carious lesions.

Diminished localization of the energy on the tissue's surface makes vaporization of soft tissue with an Nd:YAG laser slower than with better-absorbed laser wavelength tissue vaporization required a lag time until the activation point occurs (the point at which tissue begins to vaporize). To enhance surface absorption of energy and shorten lag time,

topical application of photo-absorbing black dyes to the tissue is recommended.[113]

Beside, advantages, like good homeostasis and optical fiber delivery system, Nd:YAG laser offers some disadvantages:

- Direct exposure of the pulp by Nd:YAG laser light may occur when this wavelength of energy is directed either towards crown/root of the tooth.
- Pulpal damage, such as denaturation and disruption of vascular and neuronal tissue can occur and is associated with a decreased pulpal function. Although, decreased sensitivity may be popular from patients perspective it is important to realize that laser-induced pulpal damage may require endodontic therapy, and wound healing can be delayed for few days or more.[27]

Manufacturer : Incisive

: Millennium

: Lares

Properties

1. *Active medium*: Neodymium-doped yttrium aluminum garnet.
2. *Wavelength*: 1064 nm
3. *Method of pumping*: Optical
4. *Emission mode*: Single or multimode
5. *Output power*: 1 J/pulse

2. Carbon Dioxide (CO_2) Laser

Carbon dioxide laser is one of the earliest gas lasers to be invented by **CKN Patel** of Bell Laboratories in 1964, and is still the most useful today. It is also the *highest power (10 KW) continuous wave laser* available today.[99]

CO_2 laser is the *first laser to receive FDA clearance* for oral use in 1976. It produces a beam of infrared light centering around 9.4 and 10.6 μm.[123]

CO_2 laser is a gas active medium laser that incorporates a sealed tube containing a gaseous mixture with CO_2 molecules pumped via electrical discharge current. The filling gas within the discharge tube consists primarily of:[40]

- CO_2—10 to 20%
- N_2—10 to 20%
- H_2 and/or xenon
- Helium

It is delivered through a hollow tube-like waveguide in a continuous or gated pulsed mode.[40]

The wavelength is well absorbed by water. It can easily cut and coagulate soft tissue and has a shallow depth of penetration into the tissue which is important when treating mucosal lesions. In addition, it is useful in vaporizing dense fibrous tissue.[112]

CO_2 laser was used to achieve sterilization scar formation and minimize the formation of a hematoma as it leaves residues of carbon called **Char** which when left in place it serves as a biological dressing, thus maintaining sterility (Moritz et al, 1998).[31]

CO_2 laser produces radiation which falls in the infrared region and coincides closely with some of the absorption bands of apatite (Nelson and Featherstone, 1982; Nelson and William, 1982). Therefore, tooth structure adjacent to soft tissue surgical site must be shielded from incident laser beam; usually a metal instrument placed in the sulcus provides protection.[31]

The CW emission of CO_2 laser devices limits hard tissue application because carbonization and crazing of tooth structure can occur due to the long pulse duration and low peak powers (Kawabata et al, 1998). However, research using experimental devices and short pulse shows favorable results for surface modification and strengthening of tooth enamel for increased caries resistance.[31]

Irradiation using defocused beam is recommended, because a focused beam can possibly perforate pulp tissue and cause bleeding (Shoji, Nakamura and Huriuchi, 1985).[31]

Applications

A. Soft tissue
1. Soft tissue incision and ablation
2. Gingival troughing
3. Esthetic contouring of gingiva
4. Frenectomy and gingivectomy
5. De-epithelization of gingival tissue.

B. Hard tissue
1. Treatment of dentinal hypersensitivity
2. Dental hard tissue ablation.
3. Treatment of tooth fracture
4. Prevention of dental caries as it promotes incorporation of fluoride ions into the enamel.

Advantages
1. Excellent homeostasis
2. Removes infected tissue quickly and efficiently.
3. Reduced mechanical trauma
4. Postoperative pain, swelling is minimal.
5. Reduced bacteremia
6. Contribution in dentin formation.

Disadvantages
1. Cost of the laser
2. Lack of tactile feedback since CO_2 laser is used in a non-contact mode.
3. Laser light impinges on soft tissue thus also known as *laser light knife*.
4. Black brown appearance of the treated tissues.

Properties
1. *Active medium:* Carbon dioxide and nitrogen.
2. *Wavelength:* 9.4 and 10.6 μm
3. *Method of pumping:* Electrical excitation.

4. *Mode of operation:* Pulsed or CW.

5. *Output power:* 1 to 10,000 W.

3. Argon Laser

This laser belongs to the category of noble gas ion lasers, which operates in the spectral regions of visible and ultraviolet. This laser is also known as "ion-laser" and was developed by **William Bridges** et al in 1964.[99]

About 25 different visible wavelengths can be evolved with argon-ion laser between 408.9 and 686.1 nm. They can also provide more than 10 UV wavelengths between 275 and 363 nm. *514 and 488 nm is the most commonly used emission wavelengths* to be used in dentistry.[99]

It is fiber optically delivered in continuous wave and gated-pulsed modes.[40]

The *488 nm (blue in color)* emission is the wavelength needed to activate camphoroquinone, the most commonly used initiator that causes polymerization of resin in composite restorative materials. The beam divergence of this blue light, when used in a non-contact mode produces an excessive amount of photons, thus providing curing energy. The argon can also be used with other laboratory and chairside materials, such as light-activated whitening gels and impression materials.[40]

The *514 nm (blue green in color)* wavelength has its peak absorption in tissue containing hemoglobin, hemosiderin and melanin; thus it has excellent hemostatic capabilities.[40]

Neither wavelength is well absorbed in dental hard tissue or in water. The poor absorption into enamel and dentin is advantageous when using this laser for cutting and sculpting gingival tissues because there is minimal interaction and thus minimal damage occurs to the tooth surface.[40]

Both the wavelengths can be used as an aid in caries detection. When argon laser light illuminates the tooth the diseased area appears dark orange-red in color which is easily discernible from the surrounding healthy structures.[40]

Properties[99]

1. *Gas/active medium:* Ionized argon
2. *Wavelength:* 488 to 514 nm
3. *Method of pumping:* Electrical discharge
4. *Emission mode:* Continuous wave
5. *Output power:* 100 mW to 50 W.

4. Helium–Neon Laser

Helium–Neon laser usually called *He–Ne* laser is a type of gas laser which was first demonstrated by **Ali Javan** et al of Bell Labs in 1961 using a mixture of helium and neon.[99]

Active medium of helium neon laser is a mixture of helium and neon gases in a 5:1 to 20:1 ratio contained at low pressure.[99]

It usually operates in the red region of electromagnetic spectrum at 632.8 nm.[40]

- Common application includes low-level laser therapy (LLLT) and treatment of dentin hypersensitivity.[40]

Properties[99]

1. *Active medium:* Helium and neon
2. *Wavelength:* 632.8 nm
3. *Method of pumping:* Electrical discharge
4. *Mode of operation:* CW
5. *Output power:* 0.5 to 100 mW.

5. Alexandrite Laser

Alexandrite, a transition metal, is used as a solid-state laser. It is a chrysoberyl crystal $(BeAl_2O_4)$ doped with active chromium ion (Cr^{3+}). The concentration of chromium can be up to 0.4%. The optical and mechanical properties of alexandrite are similar to ruby laser.[99]

Wavelength of this laser ranges from 700 to 820 nm.

The **salient characteristics** of alexandrite laser are:[99]

1. This laser is operated with high average power.
2. It can operate in CW as well as pulsed mode which can be Q-switched and mode locked.
3. Absorption takes place in the visible spectrum.
4. It is the only laser which can be argon and krypton ion laser.

Applications[40]

1. Selective photothermolysis
2. Removal of tattoos and pigmentation
3. Dental hard tissue ablation
4. Removal of kidney stones.

Properties[99]

1. *Active medium*: Chrysoberyl ($BeAl_2O_4$) doped with chromium ions
2. *Wavelength*: 700–820 nm
3. *Mode of operation*: Single or multimode
4. *Method of pumping*: Optical
5. *Output power*: 1.2 J per pulse.

6. Holmium: YAG Laser

Holmium: YAG laser is a solid-state laser with holmium and thulium ions doped in a solid crystal of yttrium aluminum garnet sensitized with chromium. It is fiberoptically delivered in free running pulsed mode. [40]

The wavelength produced by this laser is 2.1 µm (2100 nm) which is in the near infrared portion of invisible non-ionizing radiation spectrum. It is absorbed by water 100 times greater than Nd:YAG and is used mainly for soft tissue incision and ablation including: [40]

• Gingival troughing
• Esthetic contouring of gingiva
• Treatment of oral ulcers
• Frenectomy
• Gingivectomy

• Arthroscopic surgery.

This laser does not react with any tissue pigment or hemoglobin.

Properties[99]

1. *Active medium*: Holmium doped in a crystal of yttrium aluminum garnet.
2. *Wavelength:* 2.1 µm (2100 nm)
3. *Mode of operation*: Pulsed

7. Erbium Lasers

Dentistry has a new weapon in the fight against tooth decay. This **"Light saber of dentistry"** is the Erbium laser. These hard tissue erbium lasers have the capability to prepare enamel and dentin, remove caries, bone and cementum in addition to removing soft tissue.[51]

These lasers offer 2 distinct wavelengths but with similar properties:[51]

• **Erbium, chromium: YSGG** with a wavelength of 2780 nm, and
• **Erbium: YAG** with a wavelength of 2940 nm.
  – Both these lasers are placed in the mid-infrared, invisible and non-ionizing portion of the spectrum.
  – Studies between 1998 and 1991 by Hibst and colleagues and Keller et al showed that tooth structure could be removed by Er:YAG without causing any measurable degree of thermal damage.[57]
  – During the mid-1990s research examined the safety and value of using Er:YAG for preparation of hard tissue. In these studies, it was seen that this wavelength would ablate solid tooth structure without thermal damage.[57]
  – Although the *first* Er:YAG laser system *(KAVO Key laser, Germany)* was introduced commercially in 1992; it received FDA clearance in the United States in 1997. With this clearance came approval for

caries removal, cavity preparation and conditioning of tooth.[57]
- It is these 2 wavelengths (Er:YAG and Er, Cr:YSGG) that dominate the hard tissue laser market since 2004.[57]
- All erbium lasers shows a common characteristic, i.e. affinity for all wavelengths to be highly absorbed by water, Hydroxyapatite and collagen.[57]

Absorption Coefficient in Water and Enamel

Table 5.2 shows absorption coefficient of lasers in water and enamel.

Table 5.2: Absorption coefficient of lasers in water and enamel

	In water (absorption depth [a])	In enamel (absorption depth [a])
Er, Cr:YSGG (2.78 µm)	6500 cm⁻¹ (1.6 µm)	400 cm⁻¹ (25 µm)
Er:YAG (2.94 µm)	12,250 cm⁻¹ (0.9 µm)	800 cm⁻¹ (13 µm)

[a] Depth at which intensity falls to 1/e of initial intensity.

The Er:YAG and Er, Cr:YSGG wavelengths cannot be delivered through quartz optical fibers like soft tissue lasers (e.g. diode and Nd:YAG) can. "*Infrared fibers*" are made of materials other than quartz transmits the mid-infrared wavelengths needed to deliver the laser energy to the surgical site.[57] The quality of these fibers continues to grow from when the first lasers were introduced to dentistry in 1997. Miserendino, in an independent study published by *Manni* on the first Er:YAG laser cleared for dentistry stated that only 11% of users obtained more than 100 uses out of their fiber and 30% got 50 or more uses. [57]

Clinical Applications[51]

1. **Hard tissue** – Class I to VI cavity preparation.
   – Removal of caries

   – Hard tissue etching and roughening
   – Enameloplasty
   – Osteoplasty
   – Hard tissue ablation

2. **Soft tissue** Incision, excision, vaporization, ablation and coagulation or oral soft tissue.
   – Frenectomy, Gingivectomy and Gingivoplasty
   – Gingival troughing
   – Operculectomy
   – Hemostasis
   – Implant recovery
   – Pulpotomy and Pulpectomy
   – Crown lengthening

3. **Endodontic uses**[26]
   – Access opening, root canal preparation debridement and cleaning (*photon-induced photo-acoustic streaming, PIPS*)
   – Apicectomy
   – Root end preparation
   – Removal of pathological and hyperplastic tissue.

Advantages of Erbium Laser

Extensive studies (FDA human clinical trials) were completed that included clinical, histologic, radiographic and dye penetration of 1700 teeth. The FDA studies demonstrated the following features:

1. Pulp vitality is not compromised.
2. Tooth structure is equivalent between laser and control groups and surface morphology does not change except at treatment site.
3. There is efficiency of standard dental laser treatment and various laser wavelengths

for etching and cavity preparation (animal studies).

4. No anesthesia required due to numbing effect of the laser.
5. Multiple quadrant dentistry can be followed.
6. The laser can remove caries completely and effectively.
7. The laser can perform cavity preparation effectively.
8. The laser can etch teeth effectively.
9. The quality of cavity preparation is equivalent to that obtained with a dental handpiece.

Properties[99]

A. Er:YAG Laser

1. *Active medium:* Erbium doped in a solid crystal of yttrium.
2. *Wavelength:* 2940 nm
3. *Emission mode:* Continuous wave/pulsed
4. *Delivery system:* Optical fiber or wave-guide

B. Er, Cr:YSGG

1. *Active medium*: Erbium and chromium doped in solid crystal of yttrium scandium gallium garnet.
2. *Wavelength*: 2780 nm
3. *Emission mode*: Continuous wave/pulsed
4. *Delivery system:* Optical fiber

Recommended Power for Erbium Family of Laser[57]

A. Enamel 4–8 W
B. Dentine 2–5 W
C. Bone 1.5 –3 W
D. Soft tissue 1–3 W

8. Semiconductor/Diode/Low-level Laser

The concept of semiconductor lasers date back in 1961 when Duraffourg, Bernard, Bosov and others independently suggested the possibility of stimulated emission of photons in semiconductor materials due to transmission between conduction and valence bands.[99]

Semiconductor lasers are laser diodes which are pumped with on electrical current in a region where an n-doped and a p-doped semiconductor materials meet.[99]

The most popular lasers are relatively inexpensive diode units that were developed in early 1980s.

The **GaAs (Gallium-Arsenide, 904 nm) diode laser** was developed in early 1980s and was typically 1 to 4 mW.[123]

GaAlAs (Gallium-Aluminum-Arsenide, 780–890 nm) diode laser was developed in the late 1980s. It was originally designed as 10–30 mW unit but since in late 1990s has featured up to 500 mW.[123]

The **InGaAlP (Indium-Gallium-Aluminum phosphide, 630–700 nm) diode laser** was developed in mid-1990s. Typically 25 to 50 mW, they offer an alternative to the He–Ne laser for surface wound healing. Combination probes of laser wavelengths or more than 2 laser diodes with LEDs of various wavelengths may be used as *"Cluster probes."*[123]

In a diode laser, the active medium is sandwiched between silicon wafers (Fig. 5.1). Due

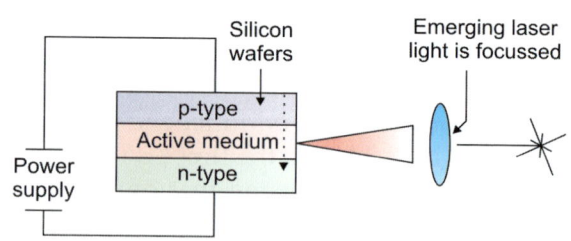

Examples of diode lasers GaAs, InGaAlP and GaAlAs.
(Ga = Gallium, As = Arsenide, In = Indium)

Fig. 5.1: Schematic outline of a typical diode laser. Optical reflective mirrors are replaced by polishing the respective ends of the crystals to enable internal reflection

to the crystalline nature of active medium, e.g. GaAlAs, it is possible to selectively polish the ends of the crystal to produce totally and partially reflective surfaces. The discharge of current from one silicone wafer to the other across the active medium releases photons from the active medium.[123]

Applications[123]

1. Treatment of dentinal hypersensitivity
2. Photosensitization
3. Wound healing
4. For relieving postsurgical pain and
5. Analgesia

Contraindications

Diode laser light is generally divergent, however, if the light is collimated the risk of eye injury increases significantly. Protective goggles specific for the wavelength must be used for the patient and the therapist.[123]

Although there are no contraindications reported for dental therapeutic laser, some caveats and side effects still exist. Because laser light affects several rheologic factors, patients with coagulation disorders need special attention. Patients with chronic pain have reported increased tiredness for a brief period and long-standing pain conditions may increase transiently.[123]

6

Lasers in Operative Dentistry

Since the past 15 years, dental lasers have had a huge growth in practical dental application for use of a variety of dental lasers. Specific laser devices are cleared by the US Food and Drug Administration (FDA) for a number of soft tissue applications, including intraoral soft tissue surgery (ablating, incising, excising, coagulating), sulcular debridement, treatment of aphthous ulcers and hepatic lesions, removal of coronal pulp and pulpectomy (adjuncts to root canal procedures) and coagulation of extraction sites.[74]

Hard tissue applications include caries removal, cavity preparation, selective caries removal in enamel, enamel roughening, tooth preparation to obtain access to root canal, root canal cleaning and root canal preparation including enlargement, apicectomy, bone cutting, shaving, contouring and resection.[74] Miscellaneous uses of lasers include curing of composite materials, removal of composite filling materials and softening of gutta-percha. Lasers are also used as an aid in diagnoses of dental caries, illumination for caries detection, endodontic orifice location and blood flow measurements.[74]

Generally, a specific laser device is maximized for diagnosis or for use in soft/hard tissues.

A. DIAGNOSTIC LASER APPLICATIONS FOR DETECTION OF DENTAL CARIES

Caries is a chronic, slowly progressive disease and the symptoms are not detected upon the onset of disease, but generally many years later (Verdenshot et al, 1999).[71] On the basis of current concepts of disease process, lesion detection and early intervention, the primary goals of modern clinical management of caries are:

- To inhibit the initiation of new lesions.
- To arrest the progression of established lesions, and
- To enhance the natural process of lesion repair by remineralization (Feather Stone 2004).[71]

For several decades, the accepted method for detecting carious lesions in patients, as well as in clinical trial has been a combination for clinical examination (visual tactile, light, mirror and probing) and bitewing radiographs. Visual inspection is based on subjective evaluations. Furthermore this method is qualitative, which restricts its applications, such as for monitoring lesion and development and controlling the effectiveness of preventive, procedures.[71] The use of dental explorer to probe enamel is no longer recommended because probing was shown to potentially damage the enamel surface of carious lesions and even cause cavitations, thereby increasing the rate of progressions of carious lesions (Ekstrand et al, 1987, Van Drop et al, 1988). Thus it is necessary and important to look for and test new objective and quantitative methods in order to aid clinicians in detecting and monitoring progressions of carious lesions on smooth surfaces.[71]

As a complement to conventional methods, several new diagnostic techniques for the purpose of detection and monitoring progression of early carious lesions have been introduced and tested.

Among these are

1. Quantitative laser fluorescence (QLF)
2. Near-infrared fluorescence (DIAGNOdent)
3. Multiphoton imaging
4. Terahertz imaging
5. Optical coherence tomography and polarization sensitive-optical coherence tomography (OCT and PS-OCT)
6. Near infrared imaging (NIR)
7. Photothermal radiometry and laser modulated luminescence (PTR and LUM)

1. Quantitative Laser/Light Fluorescence (QLF)

Fluorescence is a well-known phenomenon in science and technology. In simple terms, light at one wavelength (excitation wavelength) is absorbed by a substance and emitted as a second longer wavelength (emission wavelength, Fig. 6.1).[19] The inherent fluorescence of the material is often referred to as 'autofluorescence'. The autofluorescence phenomenon of dental hard tissue has been described by Benedict in 1928 as a means to detect dental caries.[19]

In the beginning of 1980s, laser light was used to induce autofluorescence of enamel and was employed to develop a sensitive, non-

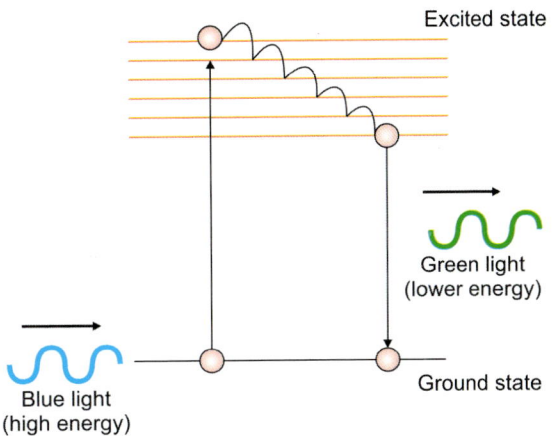

Fig. 6.1

destructive diagnostic method for detection of enamel demineralization of dental caries (Bjelkhagen et al, 1982). Since then this method has been developed, validated and applied to in vitro, in situ and in vivo studies (Hafstrom-Bjorkman et al, 1992; de Josselin de Jong et al, 1995; Emami et al, 1996; Al-Khateeb et al, 1997, 1998; Tranaeus et al, 2001).[54]

The QLF equipment comprises a light source that generates non-coherent light from xenon-lamp provided with an optical band pass filter with a peak intensity of 370 nm is order to produce violet-blue light. A CCD based digital camera and PC are also use in the equipment (Fig. 6.2). When violet-blue light illuminates the tooth surface, a digital fluorescent image is captured by the camera, transferred to the computer and displayed on a monitor simultaneously. Date is collected, stored and analyzed by custom-made software.[54]

The QLF method is based on the principle, that mineral loss, caused by destruction of tooth enamel, can be detected and measured as a decrease in fluorescence intensity when exposed to violet-blue light. The fluorescence of a carious lesions viewed by QLF is lower than that of sound tissue and thus appears as

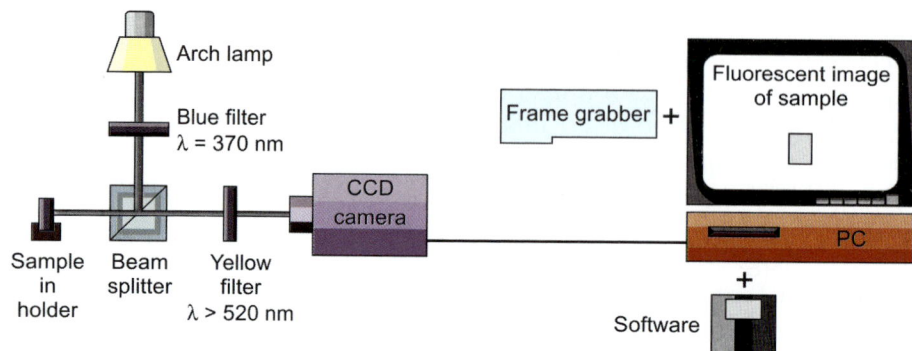

Fig. 6.2: Schematic set-up of the caries diagnostic system

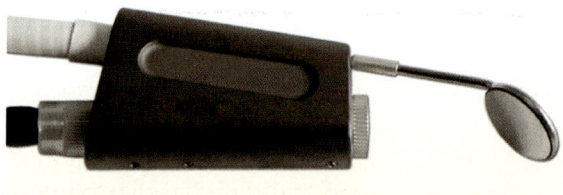

Fig. 6.3: QLF measuring head

a dark area in a QLF image (Fig. 6.3).[19] Several effects may contribute be decreased fluorescence of incipient carious lesion; the most probable are the following:

- Firstly, light scattering in a lesion which is much stronger than the sound enamel (Angmaar-Mansson and Ten Bosch, 2001) causes the light path in the lesion to be shorter than in sound enamel, thus the absorption per volume unit is small in the lesions and the fluorescence will become low.[19]

- Secondly, light scattering in the lesion acts as a barrier, blocking excitation light from reaching the underlying fluorescent dentin, and also as a barrier to fluorescent light from dentin to reaching the tooth surface.[19]

There is a relation between mineral loss and fluorescent radiance, i.e. decreasing fluorescence with increasing mineral loss (Emami et al, 1996; Al-Khateeb et al, 1997). Studies have shown that QLF is a sensitive method for detecting and monitoring carious lesions of smooth surfaces (Stookey, 2005).[54]

Advantages of QLF

1. QLF not only provides quantitative data but also displays the fluorescence image of the tooth on the monitor and this is highly instructive for demonstrating lesion progression/or regression to the patient with no danger to operator or patient.[19]

2. The depth of the lesion can be estimated to a certain extent.[54]

3. The possibility exists for diagnosis without a probe, even for occlusal surfaces.[54]

4. Designed to detect demineralized areas or lesions before cavitation and may be expected to reduce the number of hidden carious lesions that develop.[54]

Disadvantages of QLF

1. As the surface of tooth/lesion may be covered by dental plaque, calculus and/or extrinsic discolorations, professional clearing prior to QLF is essential.[19]

2. The effect of dehydration is a potential source of error for in vitro studies using QLF.[19]

3. The daylight/office light may influence the quality of QLF image.[19]

4. The method does not differentiate between active and arrested carious lesion or between carious lesions and developmental defects with lower mineral content.[19]

5. In cases of gingivitis, gum bleeding and/or increased sulcular fluid flow rate may interfere with both the capture of fluorescence images and following analysis.[19]

6. The equipment is still expensive but probably will become less expensive in the future.[19]

2. Near-infrared Fluorescence Method (DIAGNOdent)

Red light as well as infrared fluorescence radiation is less absorbed and scattered by enamel than light of shorter wavelengths so that it penetrates the tooth more deeply (Hibst et al, 2001). It is, therefore, possible to measure fluorescence from underlying carious dentin.[9]

Hibst and Gall (1998) found that red light-induced fluorescence could differentiate between sound and carious tooth tissue. Fluorescence spectroscopic investigations revealed considerable contrast between sound and carious tooth tissues when excited by a red light with a wavelength of 655 nm (Hibst et al, 2001).[9] Fluorescence was found to be more intense in carious tissue compared with sound tissue. Based on the fact, a laser-based instrument DIAGNOdent (KaVo Biberach, Germany) for the detection and quantification of carious lesions was introduced in 1998 (Konig et al, 1998; Hibst and Gall, 1998).[9]

The main unit of DIAGNOdent is connected to a hand probe by cable, with descendent and ascendant optical glass fibers (Fig. 6.4). The probe comes with 2 attachments one with the tapered tip 'A' intended for occlusal surfaces and the other with the flat tip 'B' intended for smooth surfaces.[9]

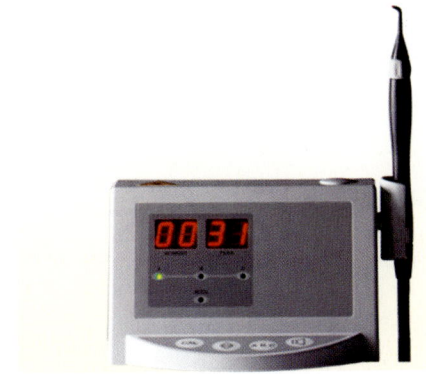

Fig. 6.4

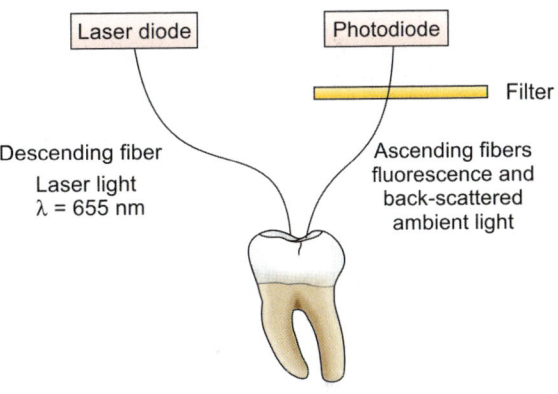

Fig. 6.5

The DIAGNOdent unit contains a laser diode (655 nm, modulated 1 mW power) as the excitation light source, and a photon diode combined with a band pass filter (transmission > 680 nm) as the detector.[9]

Laser light is generated by the main unit and transmitted through the excitation optical fiber to the tip of the handpiece. Once the tip in the contact with a tooth surface, the laser energy penetrates the tooth surface and is absorbed by the surrounding tooth material, and fluorescence within infrared spectrum occurs.[9] The emitted fluorescence as well as back-scattered ambient light is collected by the tip and carried back to a photodiode detector in the main unit via detection fibers (Fig. 6.6).

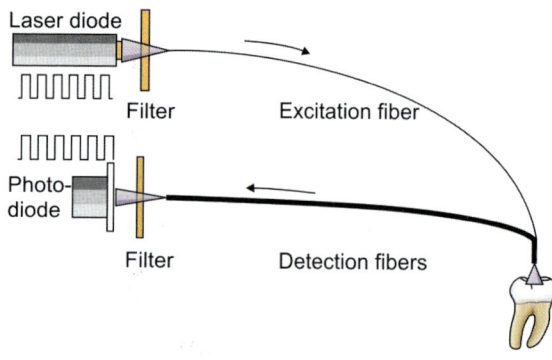

Fig. 6.6

The band pass filters absorbs the back-scattered excitation and other short wave-lengths ambient light and transmits long wavelength fluorescence radiation.[9] To eliminate the long wavelength ambient light also passing through the filter, the laser diode is modulated, and only light showing the some modulation characteristic is registered by the main unit and displayed as nominal values ranging from 0 to 99, where 0 indicated minimum and 99 maximum fluorescence.[9]

The Principle of DIAGNOdent

Hibst and Gall (1998) reported that carious tissue emits stronger fluorescence than sound tissue in the red and infrared parts of the spectrum (= 655 nm). Thus, fluorescence from a carious region, greater than that from sound tissue is expressed as a higher numerical readout by the device (Fig. 6.7). The exact mechanism of detections has not been fully clarified; however, one assumption is that the device measures fluorescence of bacterial disintegrated products within carious tissues, possibly porphyrins (Hibst et al, 2001).[9]

- 0–10 : Sound enamel
- 10–20: Surface enamel caries
- 20–30: Deeper enamel caries
- > 30: Dentinal caries

Recently, a new version of DIAGNOdent, the DIAGNOdent pen was introduced. This is also based on the same principle as the original DIAGNOdent. The main unit measures 21 cm with 2 sapphire tips: wedge-shaped and tapered-shaped. The thickness of the wedge-shaped tip is 0.4 mm with a width of 1.1 in order to improve the access to proximal surfaces, whereas the thickness of the tapered-shaped tip is 0.7 mm. The device is cordless and handy to operate (Fig. 6.8).[8]

The DIAGNOdent device has been studied extensively both in vivo and vitro for detection of carious lesions for occlusal and smooth surface caries detection (Bader and Shugars, 2004). Recent studies by Anttonen et al (2003,

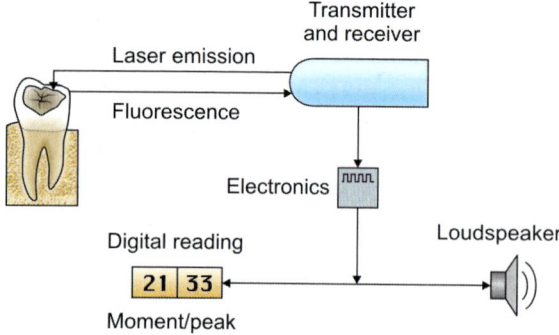

Fig. 6.7: DIAGNOdent utilizes laser light to help detect changes in tooth structure. The DIAGNOdent measures changes and displays a scale reading

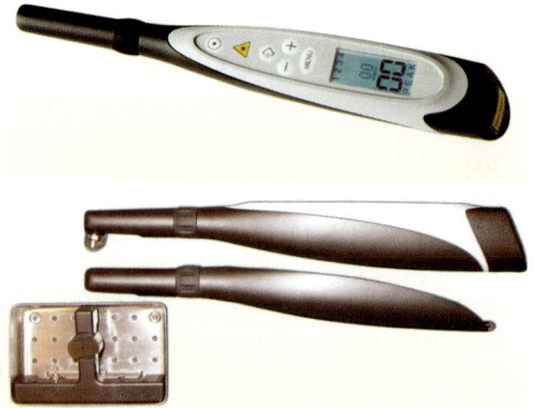

Fig. 6.8: DIAGNOdent pen and its attachments

2004) and Skold-Larsson et al (2004) support the applications of the method for detections and monitoring of fissure caries.[8]

Recently, DIAGNOdent has been tested in vitro for quantifications of lesions adjacent to fixed orthodontic appliances (Staudt et al, 2004).[8] To achieve the maximum extensions of the lesions volume, one must tilt the instrument around the measuring site with continuous rotation of the probe tip around its axis during the measuring period. This is to ensure that the tip picks up fluorescence from all directions (Fig. 6.9).[8]

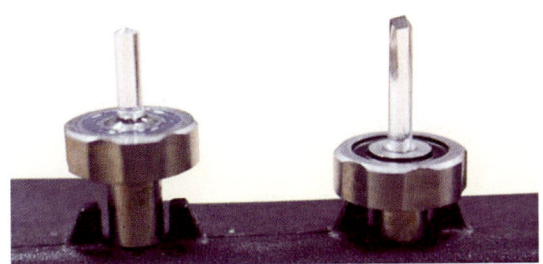

Fig. 6.9: New interchangeable tips crafted from a single piece of sapphire are at the optimal shape to transmit and collect light, giving DIAGNOdent additional applications

Factors to be taken into considerations when using DIAGNOdent

1. All measurements should be made at room temperature of about 22°C and the tooth surfaces should be dry.[8]
2. Calibration of the device against ceramics standard before the measurement sessions is important to ensure accurate measurements over an extended period of time (Karlsson et al, 2004).[8]
3. It is essential to perform the measurements on a clean tooth because the instrument is very sensitive to the presence of stains, deposits, calculus, as well as certain types of composite filling materials, and remnants of pastes which may produce fluorescence and, therefore, cause false

positive readings (Lussi et al, 1999, 2005; Shi et al, 2000).[8]

4. Potential sources of error should be considered, such as storage media for extracted teeth which may affect DIAGNOdent values under clinical conditions (Shi et al, 2001).[8]

Conclusion

DIAGNOdent is a valuable adjunct to clinical examination:[9]
- Enables better access for measuring carious lesions around orthodontic brackets.
- DIAGNOdent is best suited for caries detection around accessible smooth surfaces and occlusal surfaces.
- DIAGNOdent is a helpful aid for caries detections under circumstances where bitewing radiographs are not available.
- It is a reproducible method, with good sensitivity and specificity.
- False-positive readings can occur due to fluorescence materials or molecules.

3. Multiphoton Imaging

Caries detection systems, such as QLF, rely on the fluorescence signal observed when teeth are exposed to blue light (= 488 to 514 nm). This causes sound tooth structure to fluoresce. Carious tooth tissue may also fluoresce, but the disruption to the regular structure of the tooth at this point results in profound scattering, and no or little fluorescence is detected.[3] Consequently, sound tooth structures fluoresce at > 520 nm, whereas carious tooth tissue appears dark. It is not possible to collect light specifically from different depths within the tooth. Blue light tends to scatter substantially within carious lesions and, therefore, does not penetrate through the lesion. At high intensity, blue-light induces free-radical production and phototoxicity in the living tissue, which could injure pulp (Grikin et al, 1999).[3]

The choice of a longer wavelength of light for imaging reduces scattering, allowing the light to penetrate more deeply within the tooth. This makes the image of the tooth clearer and reduces levels of phototoxicity.[3]

In the multiphoton imaging technique, two infrared photons (with half the energy of blue photon) are absorbed simultaneously. The probability of this is low, however, by exposing the tooth to many more photos, it is possible to increase greatly the chances of two photon absorptions (probability of two-photon absorption is proportional to the square of light intensity, Fig. 6.10). This means increasing the intensity of light beam to generate heat within the tooth.[3] To generate two-photon events, a peak power of 2 KW is required. However, tooth will not be able to survive this substantial amount of power for any length of time. It is possible to reserve this difficulty by using ultra-short pulses measured in femtosecond (s) (~100 s = 100 × 10–15) of laser light to produce adequate peak laser power to increase the chances of two-photon event.[3]

Ultra-short pulses (100 s) of 850 nm laser light are generated at 200 MHz. The average beam power is in milliwatt range.[3] By scanning a focused beam, one can record from the focal place, the flourescence resulting from two-photon excitation. If the focal plane is then changed, through the enamel toward the dentin, a series of optical sections can be created with this technique, sound tooth tissue fluoresce strongly whereas carious tooth tissue fluoresces to a much lower extent (Fig. 6.11).[3]

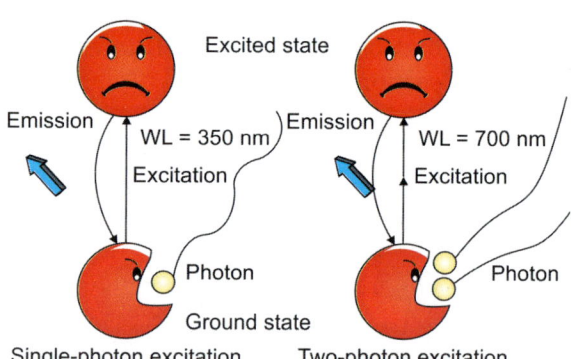

Fig. 6.11

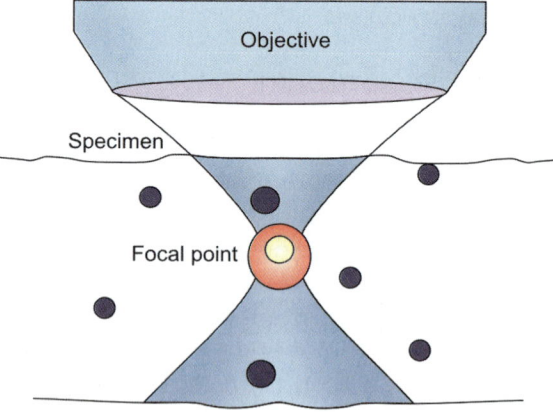

Fig. 6.12

Caries will appear darker with a bright fluorescing tooth. To highlight the diseased tissue, the image may be displayed in its negative form so that the caries appears brighter within a dark tooth.[3]

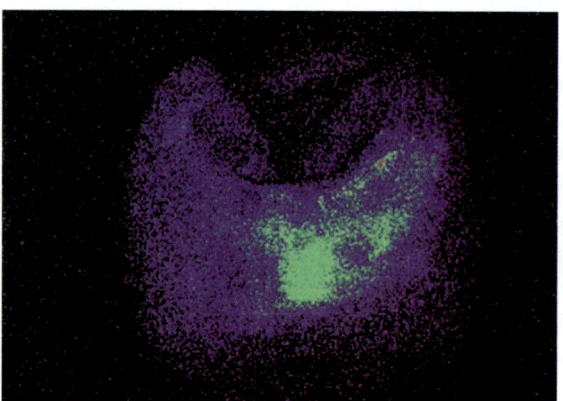

Fig. 6.10: A composite image of a caries lesion made by a multi-photon technique superimposed on a scattered light image of the tooth[3]

Advantages

1. Multiphoton imaging is able to collect information from the carious lesion up to 500 microns in depth.[3]
2. Non-invasive method of acquisitions of a quantifiable measurement of mineral loss as function of fluorescence loss, from a caries lesion in 3 dimensions.[3]
3. Low average level of laser power is used resulting in a low risk of phototoxicity to the pulp.
4. A longer incident wavelength results in enhanced depth penetration.[3]

Disadvantages

1. Currently this technique has been performed only on extracted teeth, i.e. no in vivo studies.[3]
2. Large and complex laser equipment required to produce such an image will require many years to develop into a clinically usable from.[3]
3. Only works with fluorescence imaging.[3]
4. Expensive procedure.[3]

4. Terahertz Imaging

This method of imaging uses waves with terahertz frequencies (= 1012 Hz or a wavelength of approximately 30 m). This waveform is short enough to provide reasonable resolution but long enough to prevent serious loss of signal due to scattering.[3]

For many years, no practical sources or detectors of terahertz radiation were known. The major breakthrough came in 1980s when David Auston and co-workers at Columbia University, New York, demonstrated that photoconductive emitters could be used to generate coherent picoseconds (10–12) pulses at terahertz frequencies.[37]

When a photoconductive emitter (e.g. zinc telluride) is illuminated with a sub-picosecond pulse of visible or near infrared light, electron-hole pairs are created in a semiconductor layer within the device. These charge carriers are then accelerated by a voltage.[3] The resulting transient photocurrent is proportional to this acceleration and radiates terahertz frequencies.[3] To detect terahertz radiation, photoconductive detectors can be used in addition to a technique called "free space electro-optical sampling" (EOS).[37]

For an image to be obtained by terahertz radiation, the object is placed in the path of terahertz beam alternatively, the terahertz beam can be scanned over the surface of the object (Fig. 6.13).[3] It is also possible to record terahertz images using a CCD detector. Some

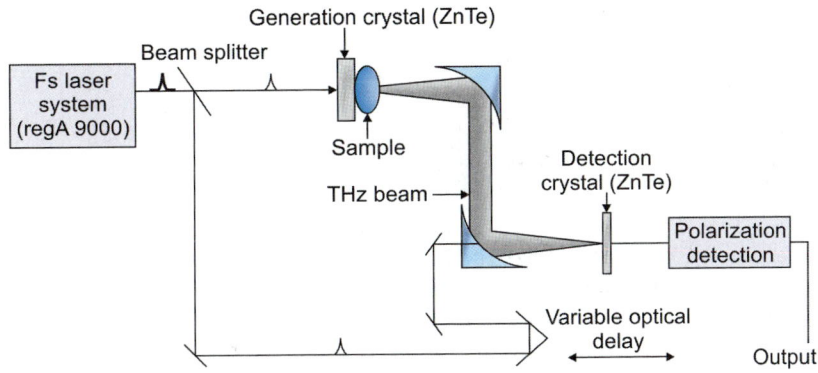

Fig. 6.13: Scheme of terahertz imaging

of the first images were reported by Hu and Nuss (1995). They demonstrated images of the inside of the silicon chip and the change in water content of a leaf over time.[3]

The application to a diseased human tissue followed. Dental applications for this technique have been limited but promising.[3]

A longitudinally hemisected sound premolar tooth has been imaged from the intact surface. Images have demonstrated the outline of the enamel–dentin junction as well as dentin–pulp interface.[3] Longitudinal sections through 3 teeth have demonstrated increased terahertz absorption by early occlusal caries, and intriguingly an apparent ability to discriminate dental caries from idiopathic enamel hypomineralization.[3] Panchromatic terahertz pulse imaging may provide a means of detecting early stages of caries. Since lesions and cavities reduce the menial content of the enamel and dentin, caries appears as regions of higher absorption in panchromatic transmission image.[37]

Advantages[3]

1. Relative transparency of oral tissues to terahertz rays.
2. Low powers used for imaging (less than 1 µW).
3. Use of non-ionizing radiation.
4. No adverse thermal effects are reported.
5. Cost of system is similar to that of MRI.
6. Both average and spectroscopic absorption can be recorded.
7. Low signal to noise ratio

Terahertz imaging could be extended to other dental applications, such as identifying periodontal disease which affects the tissue surrounding the teeth and assessing the condition of the pulp.[37] No reports indicate the time required to acquire such images.[37] Additionally, the cost of the equipment, the complexity of laser source and requirements for precise specimen manipulation with a computer-controlled X-Y stage means that it will probably take a long time for the technique to be used clinically.[3]

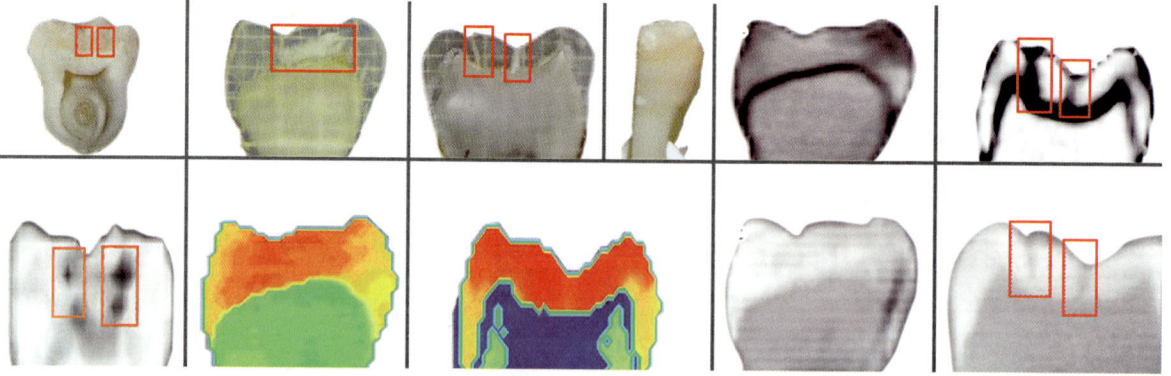

Fig. 6.14: The figures show 210 microns-thick vertical section of a human molar with hypomineralised areas. The areas highlighted by dashed boxes indicate enamel caries. An image generated by plotting the change in intensity of the terahertz pulse as it passes through the sample at different x and y values, corresponding to a map of terahertz absorption in the sample. A false colour image generated by plotting the change in time of flight of the principal terahertz peak as it passes through the sample at different x and y values. This corresponds to refractive index changes. Note that enamel and dentin are distinguished in this way

Finally, care is required in image interpretation since terahertz waves are strongly absorbed by water, a potential complication in mouth.[3]

5. Optical Coherence Tomography

Optical coherence tomography (OCT) is a picosoecond method of imaging that has been developed for transparent and semi-transparent structures.[3] Teeth fall into the latter category. It was first developed by Huang et al, in 1991 for use in ophthalmology. In the past 6 years, interest in the use of OCT for dental imaging has grown (Baumgartner et al, 2000).[3]

OCT uses light, the wavelength of which dictates scattering, and therefore, the depth of penetration.[3] Most OCT techniques described for imaging dental tissue have used wavelengths of 840–1310 nm (Everett et al, 1999; Baumgartner et al, 2000). This has resulted in imaging depth of 0.6 to 2 mm respectively.[3] Colston et al (2000) described imaging depth of less than 4 mm. The depth resolution of such system varies between 10 μm and 17 μm. OCT is based upon the principle of interference of light.[3]

When a light beam is split into two and then recombined, interference produces a pattern, the intensity of which is determined by the level of light in each beam. OCT systems use super-luminescent diodes (SLDs) as a light source. This type of source produces light with a broad range of wavelengths; each of which will produce its own interference pattern.[3] The spectral band width of light (difference between shortest and longest wavelengths produced by the illumination source) determines the depth resolution of the technique (Colston et al, 2000).[3]

The intensity of the interference is a function of the scattering caused by the changes in tissue structure of the tooth. Variation in scattering measured in relation to depth from a single point on the tooth surface is called A-scan.[3] Taking several A-scans along line produces information from a "slice" of tooth tissue, which is the tomogram.[3] The movement along the line of A-scans is known as B-scan, and according to Colston et al (2000), it takes 30–60 seconds to acquire a 1 cm long B-scan (Figs 6.15 and 6.16).

For an A-scan to be produced, light from a suitable source passes through a beam splitter

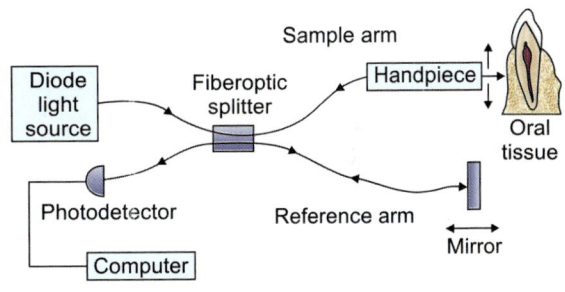

Fig. 6.15

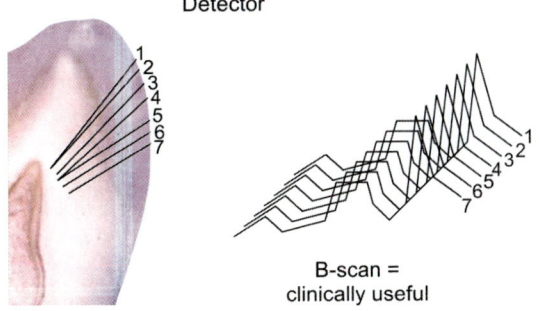

Fig. 6.16: A schematic diagram of the method by which OCT produces an A-scan and the way in which serial A-scans can be arranged to produce a tomographic slice of a tooth, known as a B-scan.[3]

to divide it into two coherent beams (wave peaks and troughs occurring at the same time) of light.[3] One beam is called the sample beam and the other, the reference beam. The sample beam goes into the tooth and will be scattered according to the nature of the tissue. Some of the sample beam will be scattered back from which it come back (back scattering) towards the beam splitter.[3] The reference beam travels to a movable mirror, where it is reflected straight back to the beam splitter. Here it is re-combined with the back-scattered sample beam. The re-combined reference and back scattered sample beams are focused on to a photodetector, where any degree of interference between the beams can be observed. In this way, changes in the scattering properties of the tooth as a function of depth can be recorded as a single point.[3]

An optical handpiece was developed for making intraoral OCT scans which provided a comfortable access to the human oral cavity and a strategy for remotely scanning the sample.[21]

OCT has been further enhanced by measurement of the changes in polarization of the beams of light as they pass through the tooth (Baumgartner et al, 2000; Colston et al, 2000) which is called **polarization-sensitive optical coherence tomography** (PS-OCT) (Fig. 6.17).[49]

A review by Wolman (1945) has stated the possibilities of selective visualization of anisotropic structures in tissue and the detection of morphological and functional changes using polarized light penetrating human tissue. Bickel et al, (1976) stated that polarization effects in scattered light too can yield information about biologic tissue. With PS-OCT, birefringence can be estimated.[21]

Intrinsic birefringence can be found in dental enamel which consists of birefringent hydroxyapatite crystals. Form birefringence is found in many biological tissues, such as collagen fibers.[21]

The PS-OCT system consists of:[34]

– A polarization maintaining (pm) optical fiber

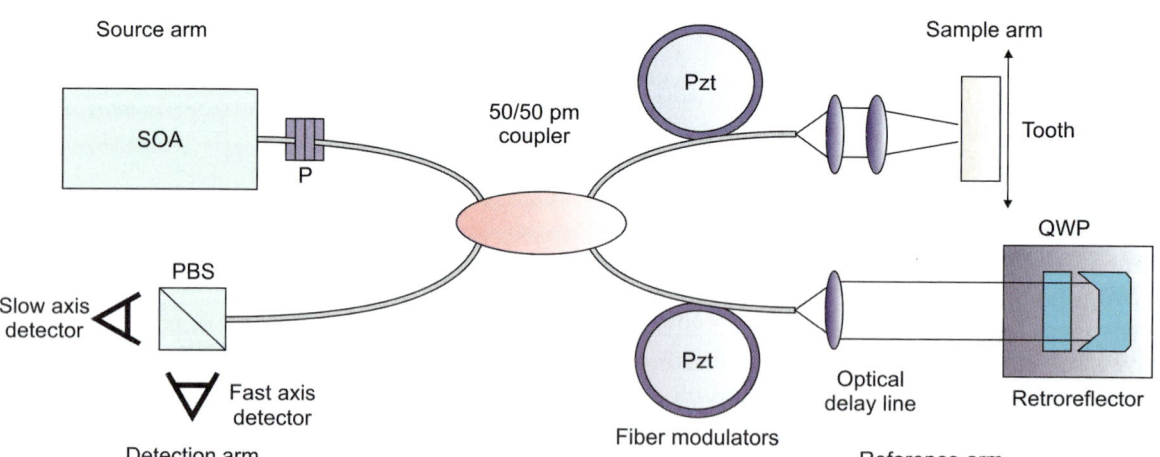

Fig. 6.17: PS-OCT system. Light from semiconductor optical amplifier (SOA) or super-luminescent diodes (SLDs) is coupled into pm fiber and split between sample and reference arms of interferometer. A piezoelectric fiber stretcher (pzt) is used to adjust the length between sample and reference arms. A polarizing beam splitter (PBS) in the detection arm splits the fast and slow axis components on to two detectors

- High-speed piezoelectric fiber stretchers
- Two InGaAs receivers to acquire images of carious lesions
- High-power (20 mW) superluminescent diodes (SLDs)
- High-speed XY scanning system for in vitro optical tomography

Advantages of PS-OCT Over Conventional OCT

PS-OCT images of sound, natural and artificial demineralized enamel, demonstrate that one can image about 1–2 mm deep sound enamel.[34]

Highly scattering structures, such as dentin at DEJ and carious dentin can be detected to a depth of 2–3 mm beneath the enamel; therefore, "hidden" dentinal caries can be detected. Longitudinal studies have demonstrated that PS-OCT can be used for monitoring erosion and demineralization.[34] The progression of artificially produced carious lesions in extracted teeth can also be monitored non-destructively. These factors are a major step in demonstrating that PS-OCT can be used track lesion progression in vivo.[34]

Other optical methods, like conventional OCT, rely on the loss of light penetration through fairly uniform lesions to estimated lesion severity, as apposed to direct measurement of the reflectivity from the lesion. This characteristic makes it difficult to apply these techniques to highly convoluted surfaces, where almost all decay is found. Moreover, using conventional OCT one cannot differentiate the strong reflectance form the tooth surface from increased reflectivity of the lesion. By exploiting, depolarization in a 1-axis of PS-OCT system, one can quantity lesion severity on highly convoluted surfaces (Figs 6.18 and 6.19).[34]

The PS-OCT system can also be used to image secondary caries under sealants and to

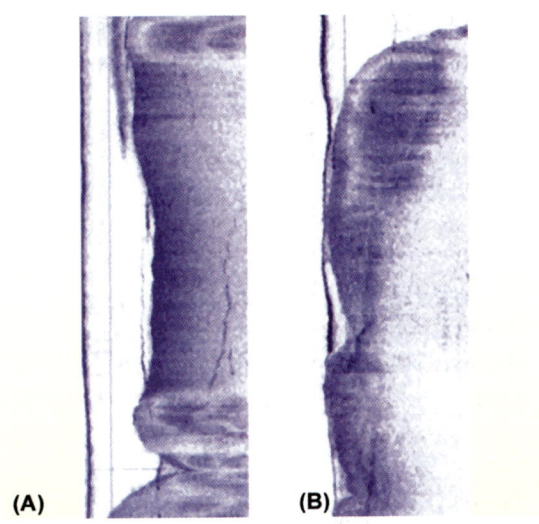

(A) **(B)**

Fig. 6.18: OCT image of dental composite restoration from the (A) occlusal surface and the (B) midfacial surface

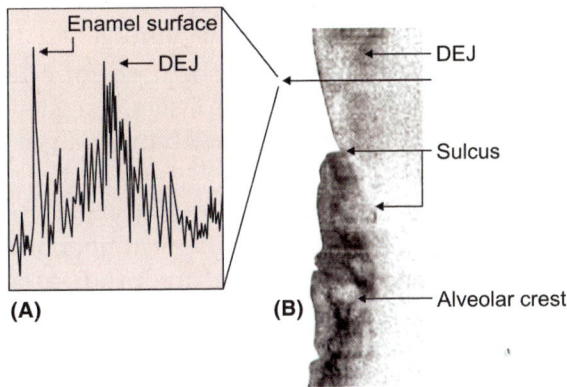

(A) **(B)**

Fig. 6.19: (A) An optical coherence tomographic image is a computer compilation of a series of axial interferometric signals. (B) The resulting image is a two-dimensional representation of optical reflections of the tissue in cross-section. DEJ: Dentino-enamel junction.

quantify lesion severity, regardless of the tooth topography.[34] The difficult task of having to deconvolve the strong surface reflection from the lesion surface can be circumvented. Moreover, recent studies suggest that polarization sensitivity can be used to differentiate between composites and tooth structures and even different composites.[34]

6.Near-Infrared (NIR) Imaging

Enamel is virtually transparent in the NIR with optical attenuation on to two orders of magnitude less than in the visible range. Transmission measurements through demineralized tissue sections at 1310 nm attenuates the laser beam by a factor of 20–25 times greater than sound enamel, therefore, NIR spectrum is ideal for imaging carious lesions.[34]

Two NIR systems can be employed to image caries. One system uses an InGaAs focal plane array that can operate from 1000 to 1600 nm whereas another system employs a low cost CCD camera that can be used for imaging at 830 nm. Images can be acquired of both simulated and natural carious lesions.[34]

Various light sources can be used for NIR imaging including NIR diode lasers, tungsten-halogen lamps and broadband super-luminescent diodes (SLDs).[34]

The SLDs provided a high-intensity uniform illumination source from an optical fiber and the high bandwidth avoided the production of laser speckle for better images.[34]

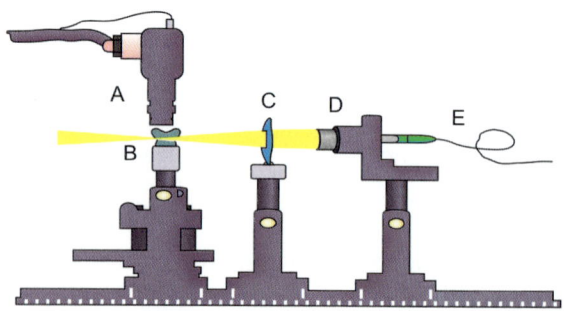

Fig. 6.20: Imaging setup: (A) InGaAs FPA with video lens, (B) tooth, (C) cylindrical lens, (D) collimator, (E) fiber-pigtail from SLD

Mechanism of Image Formation

Light from single mode fiber pigtail coupled to a 1310 nm superluminescent diode (SLD) was coupled to a 20 mm fiber collimator. The 20 mm collimated beam was focused by a 150 mm focal length cylindrical lens at a point just above DEJ which would just be above gingival margin of the tooth (Fig. 6.20).[34]

An InGaAs focal plane array (FPA) with a video lens was used to acquire all the images which were analyzed by computer software.

The enamel is transparent at 1310 nm and varies 1–3 mm in thickness. Any demineralization results in attenuation and interferes with imaging within transparent enamel areas, thus areas of demineralization appear dark as diffuse light from within tooth is attenuated.

Advantages

1. Useful for examining cracks in enamel.
2. Detects hidden carious lesions by exploiting high transparency of enamel and weak absorption of dentin.
3. The clinician is able to treat the dental decay early and effectively in a non-surgical manner.

Disadvantages

High cost of InGaAs imaging technology.

Thus, it can be concluded that NIR system can be used to differentiate among staining, developmental defects and demineralization will improve the ability of clinician to localize areas of demineralization. NIR also has a great potential for examining cracks in enamel and detect hidden lesions. Another major advantage of this method is that it enables the clinician to treat dental decay effectively in a non-surgical manner, plus the low cost NIR technology is likely to become available in the near future or an alternative system can be developed at 830/1310 nm balancing cost, sensitivity and performance.[34]

7. Laser Photothermal Radiometry and Laser Modulated Luminescence (PTR and LML)

Caries detection for a vast majority of clinicians still relies upon radiographs, explorers and visual determination. With these crude tools, clinicians are hampered in their ability to diagnose and monitor carious lesion or assess the status of a stained tooth.[110]

The first attempt to apply depth profilometric capability of frequency domain laser infrared photothermal radiometry (PTR) was reported by Mandelis and Nicolaides et al in 2000.[110]

This approach consists of a dynamic (i.e. non-static, steady state signal level) dental depth profilometric inspection technique which can provide simultaneous measurements of intensity modulated frequency domain PTR and LUM signals from defects in teeth.[110]

Mechanism

The technique is based on the modulated thermal infrared (black body/Planck radiation) response of a medium, resulting from radiation absorption and non-radiative energy conversion followed by a temperature rise. The generated signals carry subsurface information in the form of temperature depth integral.[110]

Two semiconductor lasers with wavelength 659 nm and 830 nm were used as sources for both PTR and LUM signals. A diode laser driver was used for the laser and was triggered by built in generator of the lock-in amplifier which modulates the current. The laser beam is then focused on the sample (Fig. 6.21). The modulated PTR signal from the tooth was collected and focused by two paraboidal mirrors which are rhodium coated on to a

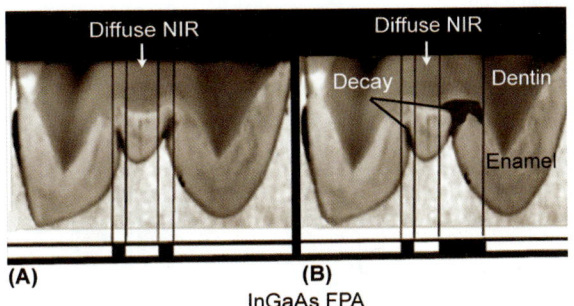

Fig. 6.21: Occlusal image contrast model, areas of occlusal decay appear darker as diffuse light from within the tooth is attenuated by occlusal caries. (A) Shallow caries in fissures, (B) caries that penetrate deep and spread in the underlying dentin may create a larger opacity on the FPA

mercury cadmium telluride (HgCdTe or MCT) detector. For simultaneous measurements of PTR and LUM signals, a germanium window was placed between mirrors so that wavelength is reflected which is then focused on the photodetector. A glass filter is placed in front of photodetector to block reflected/scattered laser light from the tooth surface.[93]

With this type of set up, two types of experiments can be performed. The first is imaging where samples are scanned at a constant frequency. The second experiment is dynamic, performed at one location on the sample. It generated depth dependent information by scanning the laser beam frequency (Fig. 6.22).[93]

Recently, PTR and LUM are used as a fast diagnostic tool to quantify sound enamel or dentin as well as subsurface cracks in human teeth (Nicolaides et al, 2000).[110] Under 488 nm laser excitation and frequencies in the range of 10 Hz to 10 kHz it was found that PTR (used alone or in combination with LUM) could be used as a sensitive depth profilometric dental probe for the diagnosis of near surface or deep subsurface carious lesions and/or monitoring enamel thickness (Jeon et al, 2004).[110]

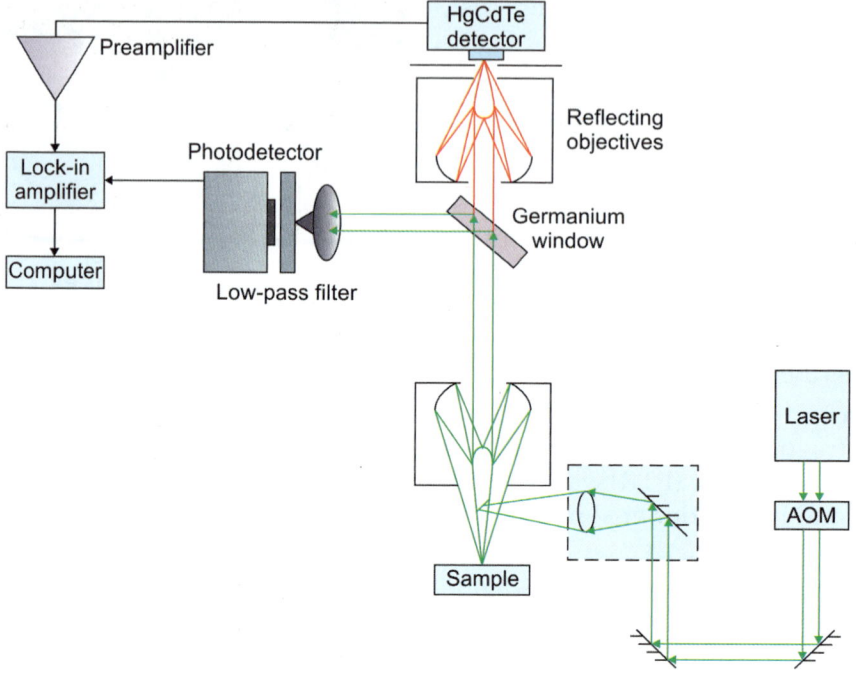

Fig. 6.22: Frequency-domain photothermal radiometric (FD-PTR) and luminescence imaging set up

Advantages

1. A major advantage is the localization of features largely due to relative insensitivity of this technique to photon scattering.[93]

2. Non-destructive, non-intrusive method for evaluating sound and defective tooth enamel.[110]

3. Much superior dynamic range of amplitude signal with regard to the defected state of dental enamel.[93]

4. Superior feature localization and resolution.[93]

5. Depth profilometric capabilities.[93]

6. Ability to detect lesions which are neither visible nor detectable with radiographs or with fluorescence (DIAGNOdent).[110]

Commercially Available as CANARY SYSTEM™

The Canary System™ (Fig. 6.23) is a device for the early detection and monitoring of tooth decay. It can detect decay on smooth enamel surfaces, root surfaces, biting surfaces, between teeth and around existing amalgam or composite fillings. It is a pain-free, safe and non-invasive early detection system.

Why the name "Canary"?

The "canary in the mineshaft" was used for centuries to protect people from undetectable hazards. Today, the word is synonymous with an early warning system or alert. Thus, early detection of dental caries allows decay to be halted or reversed using remineralization therapies.

When laser light is shone on to the tooth, the system measures the level of glow (luminescence or LUM) and heat (Photo-thermal radiometry or PTR) released from the tooth. Laser light interacts differently with healthy teeth than with decayed teeth. By varying the pulse of the laser beam, a depth profile of the tooth can be created to permit detection of decay as deep as 5 mm from the tooth surface and as small as 50 microns in size (20 times smaller than a millimeter).

Technical Specifications

Technology: Photothermal radiometry and luminescence (PTR-LUM)
Light source: Diode-laser (660 nm)
Output power: < 50 mW
Frequency: 2 Hz

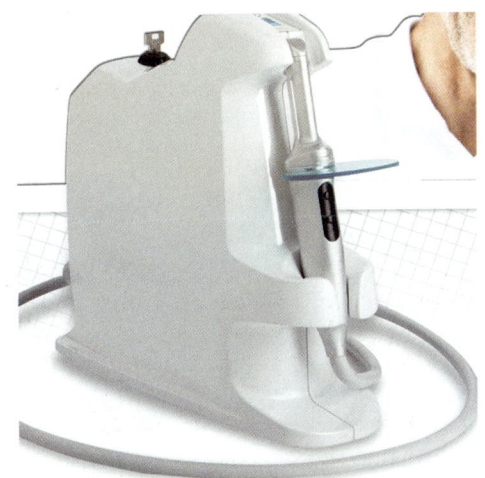

Fig. 6.23: The Canary System™

B. DIAGNOSTIC LASER APPLICATIONS USED AS RESEARCH TOOLS

1. Confocal Laser Scanning Microscopy (CLSM)

Confocal microscopy has been quite slow to be applied in dental research, even through the principle behind this technique was discovered in 1955 by Marvin Minsky (patented in 1961) and the first functional confocal microscope in a dental school was delivered in 1983 by Watson and Boyde.[129] The first commercial instrument appeared in 1987.[2]

Modern confocal microscopes can be considered as completely integrated electronic systems where optical microscope plays a central role in configuration that consists of one or more electronic detectors, a computer (for image display), processing output and storage and several laser systems combined with wavelength selection devices and a beam scanning assembly.[48]

The expression "Confocal" derives from the use of an aperture in the conjugate focal plane of an objective lens in both the illumination and imaging pathways of a microscope.[129]

Principle

CLSM is based on the principle of eliminating stray light from out of focus planes by means of confocal apertures (Fig. 6.24).[2]

Image Formation

Laser beam passes through a light source aperture and then is focused by an objective lens into a small focal volume within a fluorescent volume. A mixture of emitted fluorescent light as well as reflected laser light from the illuminated spot is then recollected by the objective lens. A beam splitter separates the light mixture by allowing only the laser light to pass through and reflecting the fluorescent light into the detection apparatus. After passing a pinhole, the fluorescent light is detected by a photomultiplier tube (PMT) transforming light into an electrical signal which is recorded by the computer.[132]

The detector aperture obstructs the light that is not coming from the focal point. The out of focus point are suppressed, most of the returning light is blocked by the pinhole. This result in sharper images compared to

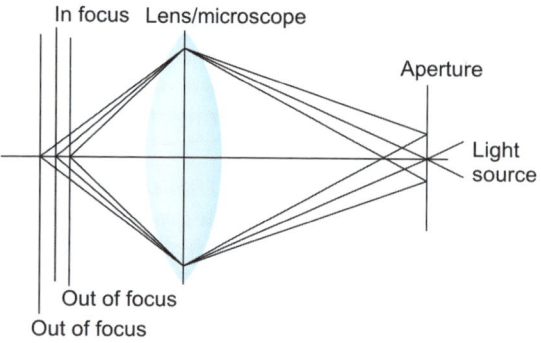

Fig. 6.24: Principle of CLSM

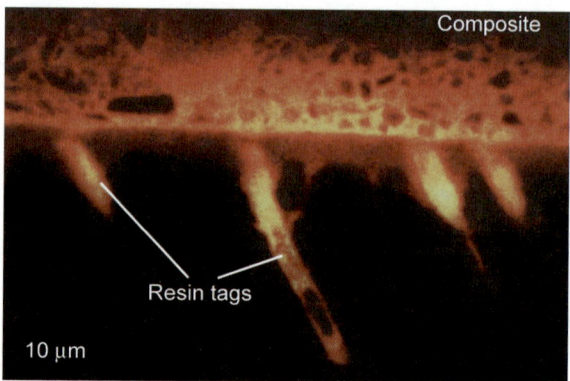

Fig. 6.25A: Bonding of composite to dentin. Fluorescence mode. The etching time was 15 sec. Both the composite and the hybrid layer are visible because of dye leaching effects or the mixing of components

conventional fluorescence microscope and permits one to obtain images of various z-axis planes of the sample.[132]

CLSM has been identified as a nondestructive tool for viewing the sub-surface tomography of enamel and dentin hard tissues. It allows real-time assessment of demineralization and remineralization processes within these tissues (Faller, Duschner).[117]

Confocal microscopy has been used to study high, speed cutting interactions (up to 3, 00,000 rpm) between burs and tooth substance below the surface of specimen. It has been also employed for pilot studies to examine the effects of lasers, such as Erbium: YAG on tooth tissue (Watson and Boyde et al, 2008).[132]

The introduction of confocal laser scanning microscopy (CLSM) has provided a valuable new technique for the visualization of bonding structures, such as hybrid layer and resin tags in dentin (Watson, 1991) (Figs 6.25A and B and 6.26).[132]

Recently, CLSM was introduced as a means of obtaining non-destructive microscopic topographies of outer subsurface areas of teeth (Watson and Duschner, 1995).[2]

CLSM is able to identify tissue-emitting fluorescent signal and has been widely used to validate the extension and removal of

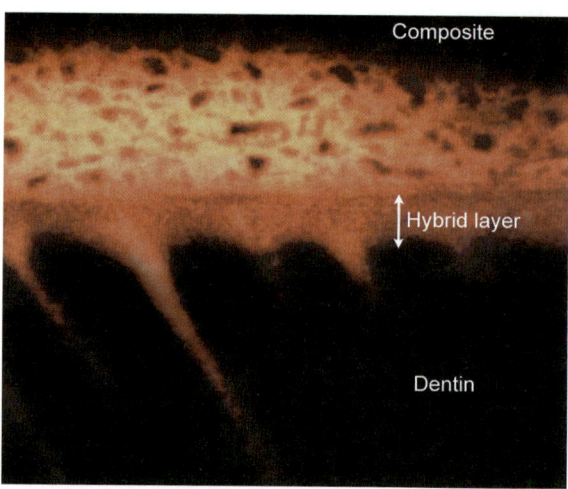

Fig. 6.25B: Bonding of composite to dentin. Fluorescence mode. The etching time was 60 sec. The thickness of the hybrid layer can be measured where the boundary of the hybrid layer is parallel to the dentin–composite junction

carious dentin which exhibits natural autofluorescence (Fabiallo Suzana et al, 2008).[48]

Confocal laser scanning microscopy also provides indirect information on the microstructure of dental hard tissue. This is mainly due to the facts that individual structures do

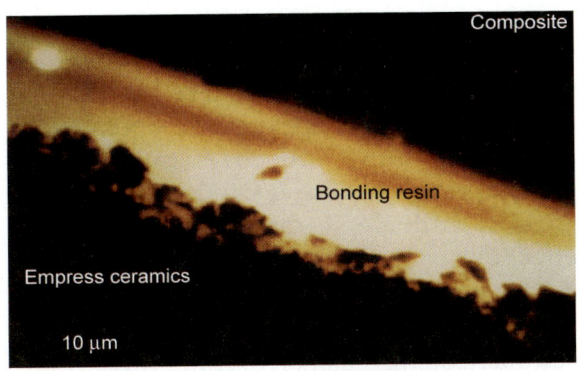

Fig. 6.26: Bonding of composite to ceramic. Fluorescence mode

not only reflect the incoming laser beam, but generate scattered light or fluorescence. Light scattering is due to organic material and to small particulate apatite mineral with anisotropic orientation. In 1995, Heinz Duschner, Adrian Lussi and Roger Walker conducted a study visualizing erosion of dental enamel by CLSM, and found that under above conditions the regularly aligned apatite crystallites in prismatic enamel appeared dark because they were translucent to the laser light.[61]

Interprismatic enamel with organic components and anisotropically aligned apatite crystallites reflects and scatters light. A clean polished enamel surface without a pellicle according to the CLSM images seemed to be relatively vulnerable to an acidic beverage, such as carbonated cola.

In CLSM, the post-erosion enamel appeared very inhomogeneous, with a widely varying degree and depth of degradation locally and from specimen to specimen.

Advantages

1. Includes a non-destructive examination, and no need of specimen during, which minimized the risk of technical artifacts.

2. The layer can be visualized up to to 100 m below the surface.
3. CLSM allows for the study of unsectioned naturally moist teeth.
4. CLSM imaging offers the opportunities to use a dye to label distinct components of bonding systems and so helps to determine what type of component is mainly responsible for the creation of resin tags and hybrid layer.
5. Provides significant improvement in lateral resolution.
6. Ability to produce blur-free images of thick specimens at various depths.

Disadvantages

One remaining problem, however, is the lack of knowledge about the true nature of the contrast mechanism responsible for interpretation under reflected light imaging (leaching ability of the dyes). Finally, the high-cost of purchasing systems often limits their implementation in selected laboratories only.

2. Spectroscopic Analysis of Tooth Structure

A. Laser-induced Breakdown Spectroscopy (LIBS)

Laser-induced breakdown spectroscopy (LIBS) is a type of atomic emission spectroscopy which utilized a highly energetic laser pulse as excitation source. LIBS can analyze any matter regardless of its physical state, be it solid, liquid or gas because all elements emit light when excited to sufficiently high temperatures, LIBS can detect all elements limited only by power of laser.[101]

LIBS operates by focusing the laser on to a small area at the surface of the specimen. When the laser is discharged, it ablates a very small amount of material, in the range of nanograms to pictograms which instantaneously generates plasma arc with temperature of about 10,000 – 20, 2000 K.[35]

At these temperatures, the ablate material dissociates (breaks down) into excited ionic and atomic species, which is observed in the ultraviolet, visible and near infrared regions of the spectrum.

An atomic spectrum is obtained by means of a spectrograph, thereby allowing elemental components of the target to be identified and using a calibration curve, quantified.[138]

Components (Fig. 6.27)

1. Laser source
2. Laser light delivery and collection system
3. Spectrometer

1. Laser Source

Laser used commonly for plasma generation is pulsed neodymium: yttrium-aluminum-garnet (Nd:YAG) solid state laser. It generates energy in the near, infrared region of the electromagnetic spectrum with a wavelength of 1064 nm with pulse duration of 7 ns generating at a power density which can exceed 1 GW cm^2.[138]

2. Laser Light Delivery and Collection System

As single fused silica optical fiber of core diameter 550 m and length 5 meter is used to deliver the laser radiation to the target material, i.e. tooth for in vivo and in vitro applications and to collect the generated plasma emission for subsequent analysis. The radiation from Nd:YAG laser was focused on the launch end of fiber which is positioned just beyond focal point of lens, via a high reflective mirror using a 250 mm converging lens.[101]

3. Spectrometer

For spectral analysis, a spectrometer is used. The spectrometer consists of either a monochromator (scanning) or a polychromator (non-scanning) and a photomultiplier or CCD detector respectively.[99]

The most common monochromator is Czerny-Turner type while the most common polychromator is Eschelle type. The Eschelle type spectrometers are used for operation in high resolutions and cover much wider spectral range, whereas Czerny-Turner type is used to disperse radiation on the CCD effectively.[99]

The polychromator spectrometer type is most commonly used in LIBS as it allows simultaneous acquisition of entire wavelength. An intensified CCD camera is coupled to a spectrometer for detection of dispersed light.[99]

The spectrometer collects electromagnetic radiation over the widest wavelengths possible (approx. 100 to 1700 nm) close to the range of a CCD detector.[101]

LIBS measurements are generally carried out in ambient air at atmospheric pressure, since the only requirement is optical access to the samples.[138]

In operative dentistry, LIBS technique is used for analysis of teeth and dental materials.[101]

Ali Saafan and Walid Tawfik (2006) carried out LIBS using portable Eschelle spectrometer equipped with CCD detector for analysis of 2 spherical dental amalgam alloy samples, and

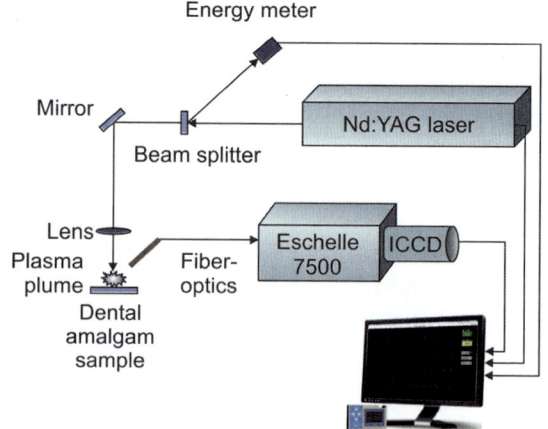

Fig. 6.27: Schematic diagram of LIBS set up

concluded that LIBS can be used for in situ monitoring and follow-up of Hg content in dental amalgam alloy.[138]

Ota Samek, Helmet H. Telle and David C.S. Beddows in 2001 concluded that LIBS is a tool for real-time in vitro and in vivo identification of carious teeth. They stated that the major constituent of tooth's crystalline enamel and dentin matrix structure is hydroxyapatite $[Ca_{10}(PO_4)_6(OH)_2]$ whose absolute abundance is distinctly different for healthy dental tissue and tissue affected by caries. For affected teeth, relative concentrations of matrix elements Ca and P decrease severely. On the other hand, non-mineralizing elements, such as zinc and organic material, increase strongly [occurrence of C193 is indicative for these].[101]

Advantages[126]

1. Non-destructive/minimally destructive and with an average power density of less than 1 watt radiated on to the specimen, so that there is no heating surrounding the ablation site.
2. Ability to depth profile a specimen.
3. Rapid-technique making it useful for high volume analysis.
4. Helps creating "elemental maps".
5. Does not utilize ionizing radiation to excite the sample, which is both penetrating and potentially carcinogenic

Disadvantages[126]

1. Limited reproducibility.
2. Variation in detection limits for sample to sample.

B. Raman Spectroscopic Analysis of Tooth Structure

Raman spectroscopy is a spectroscopic technique used to study vibrational, rotational and other low-frequency modes in a system.[99]

It relies on Raman scattering of monochromatic light, usually from a laser in the

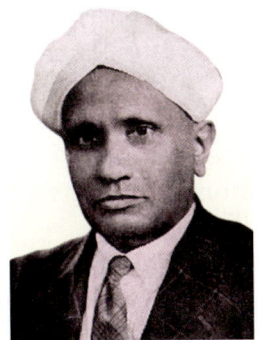

Fig. 6.28: Sir Chandrasekhara Venkata Raman (1888–1970)

visible, near-infrared or near-ultraviolet range. The laser light interacts with photons being shifted up or down. The shift in energy gives us information about photon modes and about the structures present in the sample.[98]

Named after an Indian scientist C.V. Raman (1928) (Fig. 6.28) who observed the effect of sunlight through a crossed filter to block this monochromatic light.[99]

In dentistry, Raman spectroscopic technique enables us to obtain only vibration (infrared and far-infrared) spectra of minerals by analyzing scattered light caused by monochromatic laser excitation.[62] Recently, Raman spectroscopy was applied to:

1. Detect CaF_2 formation in/on enamel
2. Study orientational characteristics of enamel
3. Identification of mineral content of tooth, and to
4. Study CO_2 laser-induced structural changes of enamel.

Advantages

1. Raman signals are emitted in the form of light scattering and can be observed from all the directions.[62]

2. An optical microscope can be incorporated easily into a Raman spectroscopic technique.[63]

3. Specimens with very low volumes (~10 mm³) can be examined.[63]

4. Simple, non-destructive sample preparation.[63]

5. Easier spectral (band) analysis.[63]

The Raman spectroscopic technique could be used much more widely in dental research, but often there is a problem of fluorescence exhibited by most biological materials when irradiated by laser. Therefore, Raman spectroscopic studies have been limited to enamel which contains only a few percent of organic material.[10]

C. Fourier Transform Infrared (FT-IR) Spectroscopy

FT-IR stands for fourier transform infrared which is the preferred method of infrared spectroscopy.

In FT-IR, IR radiation is passed through a sample. Some of the infrared radiation is absorbed by the sample and some of it is passed through (transmitted). The resulting spectrum represents molecular absorption and transmission creating a molecular fingerprint of the sample.[13]

In dentistry, particularly, it is useful for analysis of dental materials (most commonly: composite resins).

So, what information can FT-IR provide?[36]

• It can identify unknown materials
• It can determine the quality/consistency of a sample.
• It can determine the amount of components in a mixture.

Why Infrared Spectroscopy?

Infrared spectroscopy has been a workhorse technique for dental material analysis for over 70 years.

An infrared spectrum represents a fingerprint of a sample with absorption peaks which correspond to frequencies of vibrations between the bonds of atoms making up the material. Because each different material is a unique combination of atoms no two compounds produce the same infrared spectrum. Therefore, infrared spectroscopy can result in a positive identification (qualitative analysis) of every kind of dental material.[36]

Fourier transform infrared spectroscopy is preferred over other infrared spectral analysis for several reasons:[36]

1. It is a non-destructive technique.
2. It provides a precise measurement method which requires no external calibration.
3. It can collect scan every second.
4. Increased sensitivity thus allowing multiple samples to be collected and averaged together.
5. Cheaper than conventional spectrometers
6. Mechanically simple with only one moving part.

The Sample Analysis Process[36]

The Source
Infrared energy is emitted via a glowing body source. The beam passes through an aperture which controls the amount of energy present to the sample.

The Interferometer
The beam enters the interferometer where "spectral encoding" takes place. The resulting interferogram signal then exits the interferometers.

The Sample
The beam enters the sample (e.g. dental composites/dental cements) and the specific frequencies of energy which are uniquely characteristic of sample are absorbed.

The Detector

The beam finally passes to the detector for final measurement.

The Computer

The measured signal is digitized and sent to the computer where Fourier transformation takes place. The final infrared spectrum is then presented to the user for interpretation and any further manipulation.

Advantages[36]

Speed: Because all frequencies are measured simultaneously, most measurements are made in seconds. This is referred to as Felgett advantage.

Sensitivity: The detectors employed are much more sensitive, the optical output is higher, which results in much lower noise levels and fast scans enable the co-addition of several scans in order to reduce the random measurements noise to any desired level (signal averaging).

Mechanical simplicity: The moving in the interferometer is the only continuously moving part in the instrument. Thus there is a very little possibility of mechanical breakdown.

Internally calibrated: These instruments employ a He–Ne laser as an internal wavelength calibration standard (referred to as Connes advantage). These instruments are self-calibrating and never need to be calibrated by the user.

These instruments along with several others make measurements by FT-IR extremely accurate and reproducible. Thus it, is a very reliable technique for positive identification of virtually any sample. This makes FT-IR on invaluable tool for quality control for analysis of unknown contaminant.[13]

In addition, sensitivity and accuracy of FT-IR detectors, along with a wide variety of software algorithms have dramatically increased the practical use of FT-IR for quantitative analysis in dentistry.[13]

Thus, the Fourier transform infrared (FT-IR) technique has brought significant practical advantage to infrared spectroscopy and use of infrared analysis in dentistry virtually limitless.[13]

D. Attenuated Total Reflectance-Infrared (ATR-IR) Spectroscopy

Traditionally, IR spectrometers have been used to analyze solids, liquids and gases by means of transmitting IR radiation directly through the sample.[33]

Where the sample is in a liquid or solid form the intensity of the spectral features is determined by the thickness of the sample and typically this sample thickness cannot be more than a few tens of microns.[33]

Principle of ATR-IR

For the technique to be successful and requirements must be met:[33]

- The sample must be in direct contact with the ATR crystal.
- The refractive index of the crystal must be significantly greater than that of the sample or else internal reflectance will not occur—the light will be transmitted rather than internally reflected in the crystal.

ATR Accessories

When measuring solids by ATR, it is essential to ensure good optical contact between the sample and the crystal (Fig. 6.29). The accessories have devices that clamp the sample to the crystal surface and apply pressure. This works well with elastomers and other deformable materials and also with fine powders (e.g. dental cements).[33] However, the issue of solid sample/crystal contact has been overcome to a great extent with the

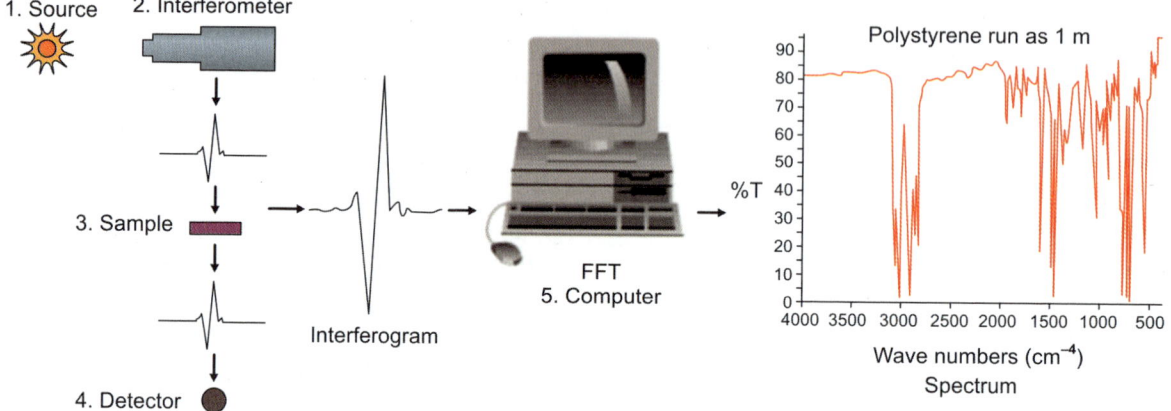

Fig. 6.29: Schematic set up of Fourier transform infrared (FT-IR) spectroscopy

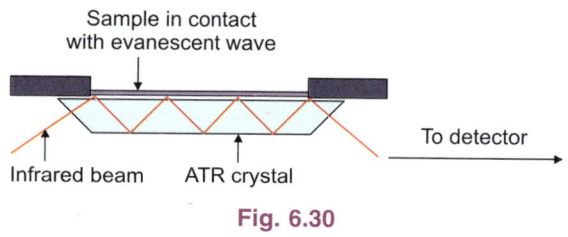

Fig. 6.30

introduction of ATR accessories with very small crystals typically about 2 mm. The most frequently used small crystal ATR material is diamond because it has best durability and chemical inertness.[33]

There are a number of crystal materials available for ATR. Crystal materials used commonly are:
• Zinc selenide (ZnSe)
• Germanium
• Diamond

Zinc Selenide

• Low cost ATR crystal material.
• Ideal for analyzing liquids, non-abrasive pastes and gels.
• Scratches easily so care should be taken

while cleaning.
• Does not work well with samples in a pH range of 5–9.

Germanium

• Much better working pH range.
• Used to analyze weak acids and alkalis.
• Highest refractive index of all ATR crystal.

Diamond

• Best ATR crystal because of its robustness and durability.
• Purchase cost is higher than that of ZnSe or Ge.
• Replacement life is minimal as life-time is higher.

The crystals are usually cleaned with water, methanol/isopropanol.[33]

Conclusion

ATR is an IR sampling technique that provides data with a best possible reproducibility of any IR sampling technique.[33] It has revolutionized IR solid liquid sampling through:
• Faster sampling

- Improving sample to sample reproducibility
- Minimizing spectral variation.

More importantly improved spectral acquisition and reproducibility associated with this technique leads to better quality data base building for more precise material verification and identification.[33]

Thus, ATR is an extremely robust and reliable technique for quantitative studies involving liquids.[33]

LASERS ON HARD TISSUES

With more than 170 million restorations placed each year worldwide, many of which could be treated using a laser, an increasing need exists for understanding hard tissue laser procedures. A more conservative, less invasive treatment of the carious lesion has intrigued researchers and clinicians for decades.

Historical Review

Investigational research into laser drilling of teeth followed a few years after the investigation of the ruby laser. Goldman et al and Stern and Sognnaes carried out the original research in the 1960s. Hard tissue treatment included caries therapy and cavity preparation. This research was followed by studies of the neodymium (Nd) and carbon dioxide (CO_2) lasers on hard tissue in the 1970s. Conventional mechanical preparation with the dental drill has been associated with fear and pain. This association may be due to the fear of the needle or the noise and vibration with the dental handpiece.

Vahl, using a ruby laser, reported extensive deep destruction of carious areas along with crater formation and melting of dentin. Kantola experimented with CO_2 laser. Cracking and disruption of enamel rods, incineration of dentinal tubule organic contents, and loss of tooth structure occurred. There was evidence of carbonization and fissuring along with increased mineralization caused by removal of organic contents. Wigdor et al reported loss of the odontoblastic cellular layer with the use of the CO\laser. Experiment with the Nd: yttrium-aluminum-garnet (YAG) laser, Lenz et al found that the tooth surfaces were sealed, and incipient caries-like lesions were inhibited. They found that an increased pulpal temperature might cause pulpal damage, if the dose is not precisely controlled. Because of the affinity if this wavelength to pigmented tissue, topical pigmented initiator was required to ablate sound dentin. Likewise, Wigdor et al showed major destruction of the odontoblastic cell layer with melting of the intertubular dentin.

Inflammatory cell infiltration debris and carbonization resulted alongside with areas of necrosis and micro-cracks. In 1974, Stern concluded that unless heat-related structural changes and damage to dentinal tissues could be reduced, laser technology could not replace the conventional dental drill. High-powered photothermal lasers are not ideal for hard tissue interactions. They compromise tooth structure and create a pathologic condition that is unfavorable. Further advances in laser technology have led to favorable biologic interactions. In 1988, Paghdiwala in the United States tested for the first time the ability of the Er:YAG laser to ablate dental hard tissues. He successfully prepared holes in the enamel and dentin with low energy. Without water-cooling, the prepared cavities showed no cracks and little or no charring, whereas the mean rise in temperature in the pulpal cavity was 43°C.

It was shown by Hibst and Keller et al that the Er:YAG laser was capable of ablating caries with negligible effects on adjacent hard and soft tissues. Keller et al in a prospective study showed that when the Er:YAG laser was used in conjunction with an adequate water spray for cooling during cavity preparation; it was comfortable alternative to conventional mechanical preparation. Relatively little pain was felt, and the procedure was thought to be efficacious and safe. Pulpal integrity was maintained. Preparation time, however, was approximately twice that of the dental handpiece. The ablation efficiency was about one order of magnitude lower than soft tissue and about a factor of 2 to 4 lower than for bone. Ablation rated in enamel was 20 to 50 μ per pulse.

In May 1997, the Er:YAG (2.94 μm) laser was cleared for marketing by the US Food and Drug Administration (FDA) after extensive scientific and clinical studies. Precise ablation of sound and carious enamel and dentin with a shallow thermal penetration depth is a quality of this laser wavelength. Likewise, a similar photoacoustic laser erbium, chromium (Er, Cr): yttrium-scandium-gallium-garnet (YSGG) at 2.79 μm has the same properties. Pulpal temperature is not increased above the threshold limit for irreversible pulpal inflammation to occur, and no charring or topical initiator is required.

Glockner et al reported that during cavity preparation with the laser, there was a temperature change after a few seconds from 37°C to 25°C to 30°C as a result of cooling with water and air. Even with trephination, there was an increase in temperature in the pulp only when the temperature-measuring probe was hit directly by the laser beam. Frentzen et al reported that the surface morphology of enamel remained rough after Er:YAG preparation. The laser treatment allowed additional etching, resulting in a micro-retentive pattern. The dentinal tubules beneath the preparation zone showed no morphological change.

Hard Tissue Laser Biophysics

Many factors must be considered when determining the biologic effects of laser light energy on dental tissue. The biophysics of hard tissue laser include the wavelength, energy density, and pulse duration of the laser radiation and the properties of the tissue, such as absorption, reflection, transmission and scattering. Absorption and transmission of laser light is primarily wavelength dependent. In the mid-infrared region of the light spectrum, the absorption properties in water and hydroxyapatite vary depending on the wavelength. Low absorption occurs at 2 μm as compared with high absorption at 3 μm and 10 μm. Absorption in water and hydroxyapatite at 1 μm is approximately 10,000 times less than at 3 μm (Fig. 6.31). The lasers cleared for marketing by the FDA (Er:YAG; Er, Cr:YSGG) can be categorized as having photomechanical effects. Laser light that is highly energetic and is short pulsed causes fast heating of dental tissue in a small area. A fast shock wave is created when the energy dissipates explosively as a volumetric

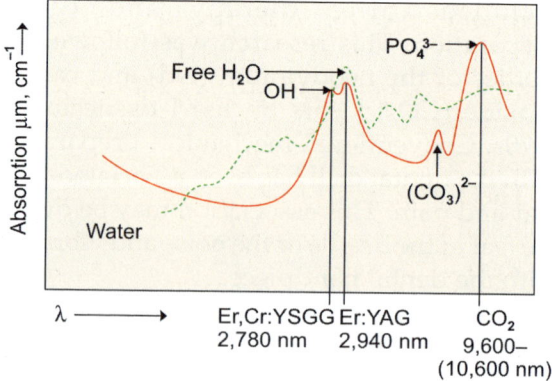

Fig. 6.31: Absorption by water and carbonated hydroxyapatite of varying infrared and far infrared laser photonic energy radiation

expansion of the water in the hard tissue occurs. This process is called cavitation. All dental hard tissue contains various amounts of water. Water molecules in the target tooth are heated, explode, and, in turn, ablate tooth structure and caries. A bactericidal effect, typical of laser-tissue interaction, occurs as well. The mechanical shock waves that occur are due to a rapid photo-vaporization of water, producing a volumetric change of state of the liquid water within the tooth. This change creates high pressures, removing and destroying selective areas of adjacent tissue. The photoacoustic effect that develops is characteristic of a short interaction time (100 μs) and a high laser density. The incident laser energy is absorbed in a thin surface layer. Water, hydroxyapatite, and collagen have an affinity for this laser energy.

The water spray of the laser handpiece accelerates this effect. Water-mediated explosive tissue removal has been shown to be most efficient way of removing tissue, while transferring minimal heat to the remaining tooth. Structural morphology of the tooth shows no evidence of cracking, fissuring, or charring. The dentin shows open tubules. Organic material is ablated, leaving inorganic components of the tooth untouched. Greater tooth surface area for enhanced bond strength is created. The depth of penetration in hard tissue is 5 μ using a 300-μs-pulse width (Fig. 6.32).

The lasers have FDA clearance to do the following:

- Remove caries
- Remove enamel
- Remove dentin
- Remove cement
- Remove composite
- Remove glass ionomer
- Ablate soft tissue with no hemostasis

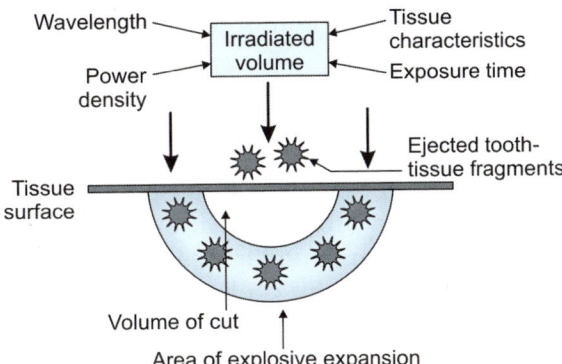

Fig. 6.32: Theoretical zone of tissue change associated with hard dental tissue exposure to laser light

1. Caries Prevention

Laser irradiation of teeth results in an interaction of light with the biological constituents of dental hard substance. If it is absorbed by specific components of dental enamel, the irradiated energy is converted directly into heat.[24] This thermal effect is regarded as being the cause of microstructure and chemical changes in dental enamel following laser irradiation and serves to explain the increase in acid resistance.[24]

After heating dental enamel between 300–400°C, a relative minimum solubility occurs in demineralization along with minimum lesion depth [Hsu et al, 1994; Sato, 1983]. Several theories have tried to explain the reduced acid solubility of dental enamel after heating.[1] In addition to reduced permeability of dental enamel following laser irradiation, the most widely accepted theory is based on the fact that bound carbonate is released when dental enamel is heated. This loss already begins following a temperature increase of 100°C, increasing to the point of almost complete carbonate loss when the melting point is reached (Oho and Morioka, 1990). A direct relationship has been demonstrated between carbonate loss in irradiated enamel and reduced acid solubility (Featherstone 1998).[1]

Another possible explanation is that free water present in dental enamel undergoes expansion as a result of heating. Both the theories are supported by the observation that the cracks run along the line of 'weaker' structures (prism boundaries).[24]

Use of an air/water cooling has a negative impact on caries preventive effect of erbium laser irradiation (Young et al, 2000).[24]

The US Food and Drug Administration approved the use of an Er:YAG laser for caries removal and cavity preparation in teeth. This was the first approval in the US for laser use on dental hard tissues. A second Er:YAG laser and an Er: YSGG laser have been cleared for similar hard tissue use. Other hard tissue uses are likely to be approved in the near future, including the use of lasers for the inhibition of progression of dental caries.[24]

In 2000, Featherstone stated that the degree of protection against caries progression provided by one time initial laser treatment were reported to be comparable to daily fluoride treatment by a fluoride dentifrice. The threshold pH for enamel dissolution was reportedly lowered from 5.5 to 4.8 and the hard tooth structure was 4 times more resistant to acid dissolution.[83]

Featherstone et al have measured thermal effects, ablation, vaporization, and thermal modeling, all at numerous wavelengths. This work has led to laboratory studies so as to establish scientific basis for the choice of laser conditions that can be used clinically for the prevention, removal, or treatment of caries lesions.[83] The underlying hypothesis for caries prevention that has now been proved is two-fold:

- There are specific sets of irradiation conditions for laser light that interact most effectively with dental hard tissues.

- Efficient conversion of light to heat as the laser light is absorbed results in increased resistance of tooth mineral to dissolution by acid.

Laboratory Studies Showing Caries Inhibition after Laser Irradiation

Studies have shown that CO_2 laser treatment of dental enamel can inhibit subsequent caries-like progression in the laboratory by up to 85%. The studies were conducted using well-established pH-cycling models that were developed on the basis of studies in the mouths of orthodontic patients. The degree of protection against caries progression provided by the one-time initial laser treatment in this model was comparable to daily fluoride treatment by a fluoride dentifrice in the same model.[28]

Mechanism of Inhibition of Caries Progression and Optimal Laser Parameters

Carbonate is lost from the carbonated apatite mineral of the tooth during specific laser irradiation. Pulsed CO_2 laser irradiation interacts with the phosphate groups in the dental mineral, is preferentially absorbed, is transformed efficiently to heat, can raise the temperature to levels that drive off the carbonate using low energies with pulses of 100 µs or less.[28] The effects depend on wavelength and pulse characteristics. By adjusting the characteristics of the laser, the optimal heating at the surface can be obtained, while maintaining the temperature rise in the pulp at a safe level of less than 4°C.[28]

Mechanically, what occurs is that the carbonated hydroxyapatite in the surface and immediate subsurface of the enamel is heated to temperatures greater than 400°C, decomposing the carbonate and leaving behind a hydroxyapatite-like mineral that is much less soluble than the original mineral, as described earlier. It has been shown that variety of conditions can be used to produce this effect.[28] The optimal wavelength in the experiments is 9.3 to 9.6 μm, with pulse durations of 100 μs or less and fluences (energy per surface area, per pulse) of less than 4J/cm². Current studies are concentrating on optimizing the laser parameters. There is no commercial laser currently available that can produce these conditions.[28]

Clinical Application of Caries Prevention by Laser Irradiation

Although it has been shown in the laboratory, using pH-cycling models, that as few as 20 pulses of 100-μs duration each can produce a similar preventive effect to daily fluoride dentifrice use, these promising results have not been tested in human mouths. It is also necessary to conduct human safety studies to confirm that the laboratory assessments regarding pulp temperature changes translate to no damage in the human mouths.[28]

Combination of Ablation and Caries Prevention

It would be desirable to develop a laser that can remove carious tissue initially and treat subsequently the walls of the area where carious tissue is removed to make them resistant to subsequent caries challenge. Fried et al have reported a CO_2 laser that removes carious tissue efficiently and can inhibit caries progression.[22] The fluences used for caries removal are higher than those necessary for caries prevention, but the residual energy may be sufficient to provide caries inhibition in the cavity preparation walls. The laser treatment would be followed by placement of a composite resin and inhibit subsequent caries around that restoration.[22]

Conclusion

Irradiation of dental enamel by specific wavelengths and fluences of CO_2 laser light beneficially alters the chemical composition of the crystals, decomposing the carbonate component, markedly reducing the acid reactivity of the mineral. Efficient conversion of light to heat in the outer few micrometers of enamel increases the resistance of the mineral to acid, if a critical threshold temperature is reached.[28] This surface alteration has marked effect in inhibition of subsurface caries progression. The author's group has proved their initial hypothesis that specific wavelength irradiation is absorbed by the mineral and converted efficiently to heat at the surface, causing thermal composition of the enamel crystals to a less soluble form.[28]

2. Caries Removal

Caries removal has conventionally been performed using mechanical cutting and drilling systems. However, these methods have some major disadvantages, like induction of pain, since it was demonstrated that in vitro caries removal was possible using Ruby laser, numerous researchers have investigated the effect of other laser including argon, CO_2 or Nd:YAG laser.[83] However, irradiation produced by these lasers had major thermal side effects, such as melting, cracking of enamel/dentin and an increase in pulpal temperature, because these lasers require a relatively higher energy density to vaporize hard tissues (Fig. 6.33).[83]

Recently, effective ablation of dental hard tissues using Er:YAG laser has been reported.[83] However, Richman et al (1998) found that selective ablation of carious dentin is difficult with Er:YAG laser. The ablation thresholds of healthy dentin and carious dentin are different. The ablation threshold of

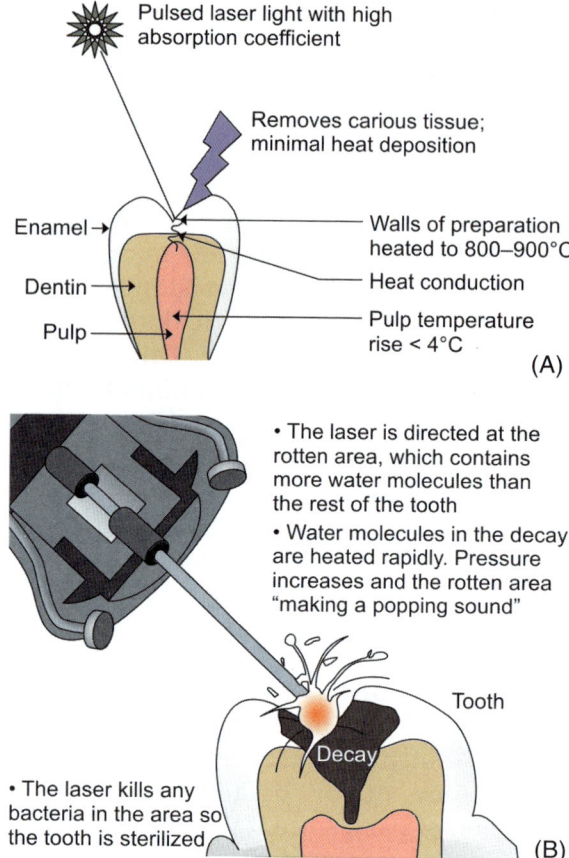

Pulsed laser light with high absorption coefficient

Removes carious tissue; minimal heat deposition

Enamel →

Dentin →

Pulp →

Walls of preparation heated to 800–900°C

Heat conduction

Pulp temperature rise < 4°C

(A)

• The laser is directed at the rotten area, which contains more water molecules than the rest of the tooth

• Water molecules in the decay are heated rapidly. Pressure increases and the rotten area "making a popping sound"

Tooth

Decay

• The laser kills any bacteria in the area so the tooth is sterilized

(B)

Fig. 6.33: Mechanism of caries removal by laser

healthy dentin is 2 times higher than the corresponding threshold of carious dentin.[1]

Therefore, very small fluences [energy (joules)/area (cm^2)] of Er:YAG laser energy is required to selectively ablate carious dentin. This low fluence will result in low efficiency of ablation process (Sheigtani, 2002).[1] In other in vitro study, investigating the effectiveness of caries removal by Er:YAG, it was found that Er:YAG laser ablated carious dentin effectively with minimal thermal damage to the surrounding intact dentin (Aoki and Ishikawa et al, 1998). The laser removed infected and softened carious dentin to the same degree as bur treatment.[1]

In addition, a lower degree of vibration was noted with Er:YAG laser treatment.[1]

Yamada, Hossain, Suzuki, et al (2001)[122] investigated the effectiveness of caries removal by using an Er:YAG laser irradiation with and without Carisolv, in vitro. DIAGNOdent carefully assessed the cavity. Their results revealed that application of Carisolv followed by Er:YAG laser irradiation at 100–140 mJ pulse energy effectively removed dentin caries; it was found that the cavity surface treated with the laser revealed various patterns of micro-irregularity, often accompanied by microfissure propagation. There was also no smear layer. The study revealed that Er:YAG laser and Carisolv could provide an alternative technique for caries removal for conventional mechanical drilling and cutting.

3. Cavity Preparation

Cavity preparation by Er:YAG laser was first reported by Keller et al in 1988. This laser was further developed in Japan, the United States and Germany and has been used not only on hard tissues but also on soft tissues.[83]

Er:YAG was successfully used to prepare holes in enamel and dentin with 'low fluences' [energy (mJ)/unit area (cm^2)]. Even without water cooling (Burkes et al, 1992), the prepared cavities showed no cracks and low or no charring, while the mean temperature rise of the pulp cavity was about 4.3°C (Rechmann et al, 1988). In 1989, it was demonstrated that Er:YAG laser produced cavities in enamel and dentin without major side effects.[1] Dentin and enamel removal was very effective at lower thresholds with no risk to pulp (Armengol, 2000; Cavalantii, 2003) and the ablation rates in enamel were stated to be in the range of 20–50 m/pulse and in dentin were reported to be as high at lower fluences.[1]

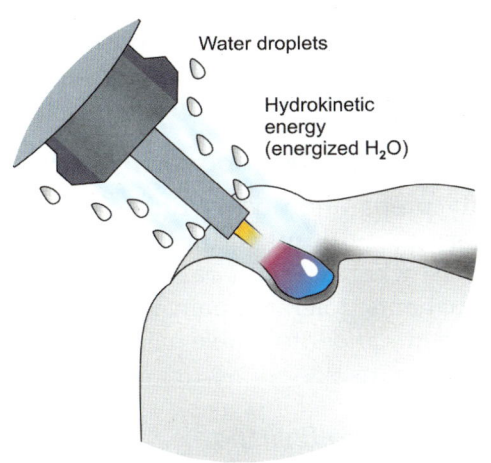

Water droplets

Hydrokinetic
energy
(energized H₂O)

Fig. 6.34

Another device that emits a comparable wavelength to Er:YAG laser is the **laser-powered hydrokinetic system (LPHKS).**[68]

Proposed Mechanism of LPHKS

Er, Cr:YSGG pulsed laser source delivers photons into an air–water spray matrix with resultant micro-explosive forces on H_2O droplets. This process is hypothesized to contribute significantly to mechanism of hard tissue cutting. The LPHKS with its accompanying air–water spray has been shown to cut enamel dentin, cementum and bone efficiently and cleanly without deleterious thermal effects on dental pulp.[68]

LPHKS Operating Parameters

The LPHKS uses an Er, Cr:YSGG (Erbium, chromium: yttrium scandium gallium garnet) crystal with photon emission wavelength of 2.78 micrometers. The photons are delivered through a fiberoptic cable and then are focused through a contra-angled handpiece bearing a sapphire tip.[68]

This tip is bathed in an adjustable air–water spray. The LPHKS device (Millennium System, BioLase Technology, Inc.) has been

cleared by U.S. FDA for cavity preparation on adult teeth.[68]

Operating Parameters of the Laser-powered Hydrokinetic System

Laser source	: Erbium, chromium yttrium scandium gallium garnet (Er, Cr:YSGG)
Wavelength	: 2.78 micrmometers
Pulse duration	: 140 microsconds
Repetition rate	: 20 Hertz
Power output range	: 0.0 to 0.6 watts
Pulse energy	: 0 to 300 mJ/pulse
Delivery	: Fiberoptic system to a terminal 750 micrometer, diameter sapphire tip with adjustable air–water spray delivered through handpiece
Energy density/pulse	: 0.0 to 68.02 joules per square centimeter

The wavelength of this laser device is absorbed maximally by H_2O molecules and also may target the hydroxyl group in enamel and dentin. Photons are emitted at various levels regulated by operator. The energy density and fluence at the tissue interface are directly proportional to the power setting. Effective hard tissue cutting is achieved at 1–1.5 mm from the sapphire tip. Defocusing beyond 2 mm from the tissue surface mitigates the cutting effect thus the distance between the fiber tip and tissue inherently regulates the cutting efficacy.[68]

Recently in 2004, a high-power Er:YAG laser was developed by DEKA (Italy), SMART 294 OD. Using this high power Er:YAG laser, class I and II cavities can be prepared in minutes.[83]

Dental pulp response to cavity preparation: No problems have been reported with respect to pulpal response after cavity preparation with Er:YAG laser, if cavity preparation is carried out under sufficient H_2O supply. In addition, the pulpal response to

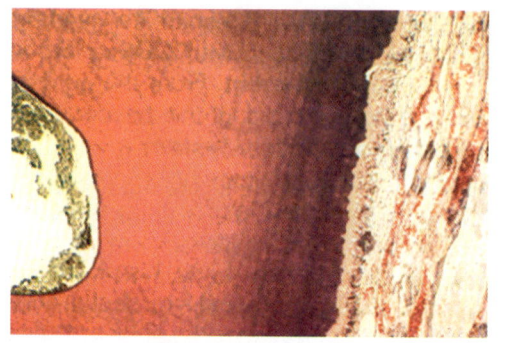

Fig. 6.35A: Er:YAG laser cavity preparation in dentin (hematoxylin and eosin)

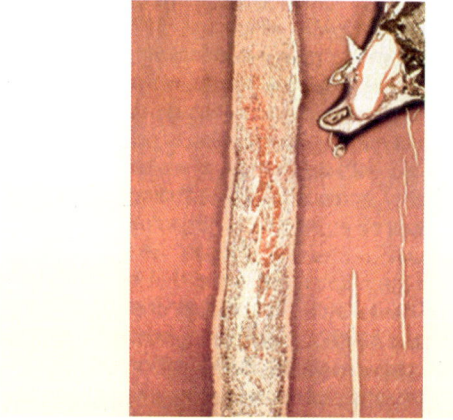

Fig. 6.35B: Carbon dioxide laser cavity preparation in dog tooth (hematoxylin and eosin)

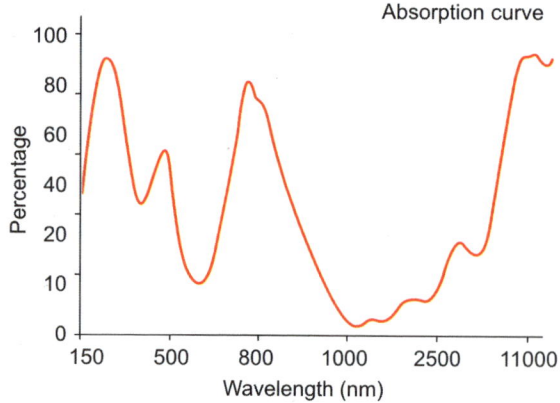

Fig. 6.35 (C): Absorption spectrum for enamel from 150 to 11,000 nm

Er:YAG laser after accidental exposure of pulp during cavity preparation demonstrated good healing capacity with formation of dentin bridge and reparative dentin (Fig. 6.35).[83]

Pain during Cavity Preparation

Cavity preparation using Er:YAG laser was performed without inducing pain in 68% patients, whereas slight pain was reported in 22% patients, tolerable pain was reported in 4% patients and intolerable pain was reported in 6% patients.[83]

Treatment Time Until the End of Cavity Preparation

Results of a clinical study by Matsumoto in 2004, the time required for cavity preparation was found to be related to cavity size as follows:[83]

Class I	:	10 to 15 minutes
Class II	:	13 to 20 minutes
Class III	:	1 to 3 minutes
Class IV	:	2 to 5 minutes
Class V	:	30 sec to 3 minutes

Perforation/exposure of pulp: 5 seconds at 7 watts and 15 hertz.

Morphology of Cavity Margin and Wall after Cavity Preparation

Er:YAG laser irradiation produced different morphological features after cavity preparation:

Visual inspection: The shade or color on surfaces treated with Er:YAG laser indicated a white, undulating surface.[83]

Light microscopy and SEM: The cavity margin wall showed a smooth, clear prepared surface, but in some cases an uneven rough cavity and surface was observed.[83]

TEM (Fig. 6.36): Lased dentin presented 3 zones. The uppermost zone characterized by

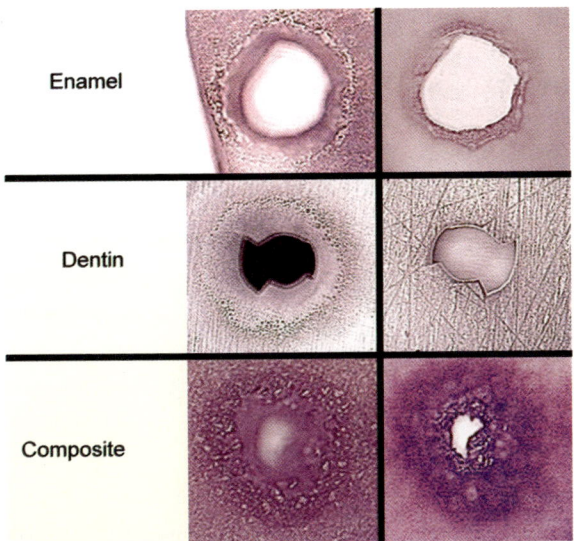

Enamel

Dentin

Composite

Fig. 6.36: Transverse electron microscopic images of lased dentin

zone of complete ablation revealed irregular microparticles of 0.5 m in diameter underneath this structure, an ablation zone of mineral components and an unaffected zone in which intertubular dentin appeared intact were observed.[83]

Atomic analysis: Revealed that quantities of Ca^{++} and P were significantly greater in the irradiated area compared to non-irradiated area.[83]

Thus, LPHKS and DEKA system is an efficient, effective, precise and safe device for removal of caries and for the preparation of tooth structure for placement of dental restorative resin.[83] It offers an alternative to the vibratory and auditory irritation that attends conventional air turbine dental bur.[83]

4. Laser Analgesia

Over the past few years, use of infrared lasers (i.e. Er:YAG and Er: YSGG) for caries removal and cavity preparation has become common in clinical practice. These lasers also contribute to positive patient experience with reduced

need for injected local anesthesia for restorative dentistry. These lasers along with Nd:YAG laser also contributes to reduced nociceptive (pain) response compared with conventional instruments, such as air-turbine drills.[89]

Clinical Applications of Laser-induced Analgesia

1. Deliberate pre-emptive analgesia, i.e. analgesia at the start of procedure can be created by subablative laser pulses to the crowns of teeth, for removal of amalgam and composite restorations using an air turbine handpiece.[89]

   [*Note:* IR laser radiation will not pass through, but will be absorbed in dental amalgam and thus dental amalgam should not be lased. The same is true for composite restorations.]

2. Soft tissue procedures: Recent studies by Zeredo et al scientifically validated use of pulsed infrared laser (Nd:YAG, Er:YAG and Er, Cr:YSGG) in minor oral surgical procedures, such as gingivoplasty, cavity preparation, gingivectomy, and frenectomy.[89]

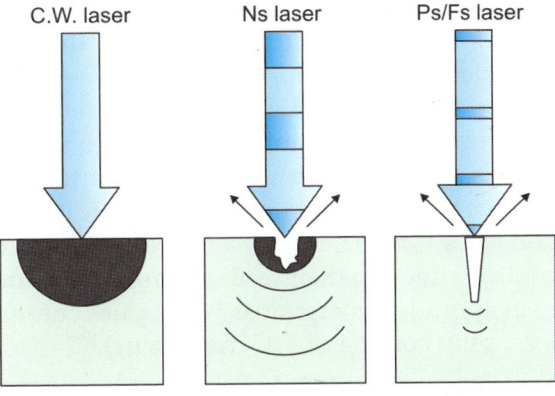

Fig. 6.37: Shock waves generated during laser analgesia

A Direct Analgesic Action

After application of laser pulses, many patients may experience slight, intermittent sensations of coolness (from cooling effect of water evaporation) and subtle "earthquake sensations" from shock waves (Fig. 6.37).[89]

There is an intriguing possibility that there is a direct analgesic effect by reversibly blocking nerve transmission. Early work in 1990 and with FRP-Nd:YAG laser showed that the pulsed laser radiation could penetrate dentin and reach pulp and was responsible for desensitizing effect when applied to cervical dentin.[89] Subsequent studies of laser-induced analgesia with FRP-Nd:YAG and Er:YAG lasers by Orchardson and Zeredo groups respectively showed conclusively that blockage of neuronal activity and a corresponding increase in pain threshold of teeth did occur after laser irradiation. Analgesic mechanisms also with infrared lasers have been attributed to inhibited release of inflammatory mediators as well as blocked depolarization of nociceptive afferents.[89]

Clinically, the blockade generated with shorter exposures (30 seconds) is more selective for depolarization of A fibers (which gives rise to sensations of rapid, sharp, well localized pain), than C fibers which explains why some patients notice low-level shock waves ("mini-earthquakes") but do not experience discomfort. Laser analgesia is known to be induced at subablative settings, which allow penetration of both teeth and soft tissues (e.g. through the pulp via attached gingiva and alveolar bone).[89] Because of some persisting C fiber activity, some patients notice cooling effects in their teeth during lasing due to evaporative energy loss (with a net energy loss, pulp cooling of 7°C may occur).[89]

Microscopic studies on both animals and humans have shown that laser-induced analgesic effect is molecular rather than histological nature. The work by Orchardson and colleagues has shown that pulsed infrared (Nd:YAG and Er:YAG) laser treatment never blocks nerve conduction, indicating that a direct effect of laser pulses on neural tissue may be important mechanism.[89]

Advantages of Laser Analgesia

1. Lower annoyance factor
2. Lowered patient anxiety
3. Elevated pain threshold
4. Short pulse duration
5. Lack of tactile force
6. Reduced pulp temperature
7. Reduced nerve transmission

Laser-induced analgesia likely results from combination of local bioresonance effect which blocks nerve impulse transmissions from some nociceptors, in combination with some gate control and centrally with altered patient responses from reduced level of anxiety.[89]

5. Laser Ablation

Lasers can remove tissue by a non-contact process, as well as guarantee faster healing and reduced risk of infection; they offer the promise of painless dentistry by replacing mechanical drills (McNally et al, 1999).[14] There are a wide variety of lasers for use in ablation in dentistry, including excimer lasers, diode lasers, erbium lasers, CO_2 lasers, etc. [14] Minimizing heat accumulation is the main factor limiting the rate of ablation.

a. Ablation with UV Light using an Excimer Laser

The UV laser provides ultraviolet pulses to some areas of the tooth. The other laser provides output radiation pulses which pass through the mirror and then through the optical fiber for delivery to the region of plume emanating from the ablated area (Fig. 6.38).[14]

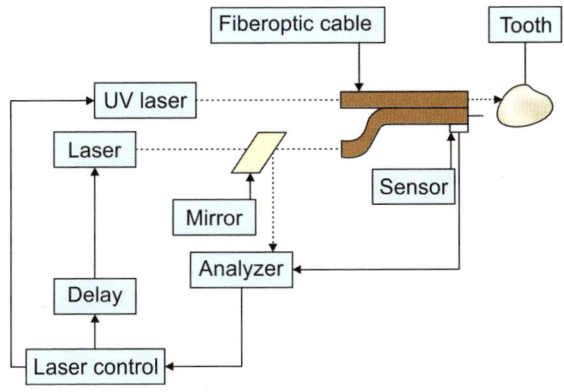

Fig. 6.38: Schematic diagram of a dental tool to deliver ultraviolet light using a laser, Goodman et al, 1999

Depending upon the material being ablated, different strengths of orange colour will appear, providing different wavelengths back into the fiber. This return signal reflects from the mirror to the analyzer. Depending upon the color signature of the plume, a signal is provided to the laser output control unit. This provides a signal to the laser in order to adjust its output power, repetition rate, etc. in accordance with the type of material to be ablated.[14]

b. Ultrashort Pulse Lasers (USPLs) Ablation

The USPLs are lasers with pulse duration ranging from 100 femtoseconds to 500 picoseconds, with power densities above 1011 W/cm² in solids (Niemz, 2004). The main characteristics of these complex systems (Freitas et al, 2010) are the very low pulse duration and the high precision that can be acquired due to the extremely small focalization area, in which a peak power up to 1.5 TW (Freitas et al, 2010) can be obtained. Also, these lasers can operate at repetition rates higher than 15 kHz and energy per pulse of hundreds of µJ (Wieger et al, 2006). In this way, these lasers offer the advantage of promoting precise smooth ablation without a heat affected zone, effects that cannot be

controlled when using lasers with pulse duration of µs or ns.

$$1 \text{ ps} = 0–12s$$
$$1 \text{ fs} = 10–15s$$

The USPLs are solid-state lasers, such as Nd:YLF, Ti:Al$_2$O$_3$, Cr:LiSAF (Alexandrite), Cr:BeAl$_2$O$_4$, Cr:LiSGaF, Cn:LiCAF, Cr:YAG, Ti:Al$_2$O$_3$/Nd:glass, and Er:glass. These lasers interact with the tissues by a mechanism called plasma-induced ablation or plasma-mediated ablation, in which the phenomenon of optical breakdown occurs. In a few words, the ablation is caused by plasma ionization, in which laser irradiation produces an extremely high electric field that forces the ionization of the molecules and atoms, promoting a breakdown and, then, the ablation or ejection of target tissue (Niemz, 2004). The generated free electrons are further accelerated by the absorption of incident light. On their way through plasma, they collide with other atoms and transfer a quantum of energy to them. This process is called *impact ionization*. During the cutting, it is possible to observe the formation of a bright plasma spark, and a typical low noise, characteristic of plasma formation.

Non-resonant ultrashort laser pulses (less than 1ps) are used for ablation, causing dielectric breakdown and consequently plasma formation, particle ejection and shock-wave propagation inside the tooth. Non-resonant interaction avoids energy deposition thus making it a non-damaging technique. Because femtosecond pulses are so short, heat conduction effects are virtually eliminated (Fig. 6.39).[14]

Serbin et al in 2000 showed that crack free generation of cavities can be accomplished using a femtosecond laser. This is not possible with mechanical drills or other lasers which generate micro-cracks that could be starting points for new carious attacks.[14]

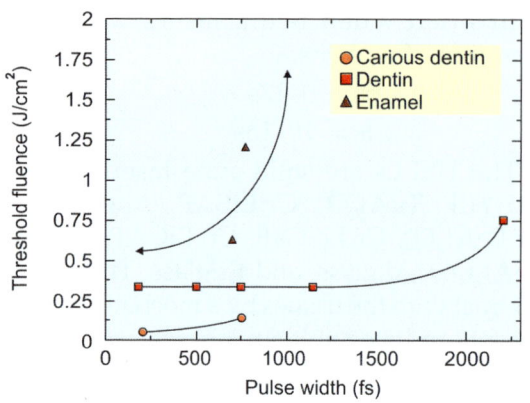

Fig. 6.39: Dependence of ablation threshold on pulse width of laser pulses

Figure 6.40 shows SEM images of Ti: Sa femtosecond laser and a Q-switched Er:YAG laser. Since the femtosecond laser is independent of material properties, it gave rise to precise structuring. In comparison, Er:YAG irradiation caused fragments of dentin to shoot out due to water vaporization, thus leaving the surface very rough.[14]

Advantages

1. Promote precise and smooth ablation without heat affected zone.
2. Decreased energy density to ablate the material.
3. Minimal mechanical and thermal damage to extremely short laser pulses.

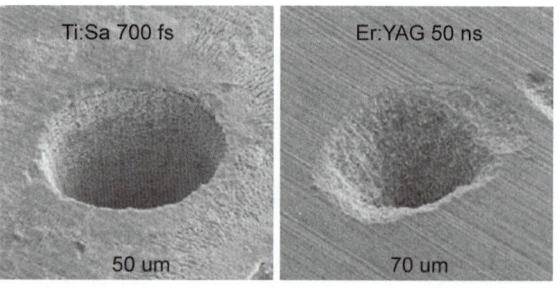

Fig. 6.40: Holes ablated in human dentin using femtosecond pulses at 780 nm and ns pulses at 2.94 μm

4. Minimal dependence on tissue composition.
5. Low noise levels as compared to high-speed burs.
6. Ability to texture surface and precise spatial control.
7. These lasers can remove any kind of restorative material including amalgam which is not possible with other lasers due to reflection of light or overheating of material.
8. Promising tool for selective removal of caries.

Disadvantages

Size, the sensitivity to environment and high cost are their biggest limitations.

c. Er:YAG Laser Ablation

It is selected because of wavelength matching with vibrational absorption of water molecules in the tooth. The Er:YAG laser uses fiberoptics to transmit pulsed laser light with a wavelength of 2.94 m.[14] The handpiece focuses a beam of about 12–15 mm from the head and depth of field for effective tooth ablation is between 10 to 20 mm.[14] Focusing is aided by a visible red He–Ne laser beam. Generally, a frequency of 2 to 3 pulse/second is used, with each pulse ablating a clean crater about the size and shape of a pinhead in enamel, accompanied by a soft, popping noise. The Er:YAG laser can also be used in soft tissue surgery, like gingivectomy or frenectomy.[14]

Use of water spray during ablation of hard dental tissue is strongly recommended to avoid temperature build-up and prevent desiccation of tissue and subsequent decrease in ablation efficacy.[14]

Advantages

1. Non-contact treatment without any unpleasant vibrations.

2. Dentinal structures are preserved and dentinal tubules are opened.

3. Retentive surface for food adhesion is obtained.

4. Painless treatment that requires no anesthesia.

d. Dye-Assisted Laser Ablation (DALA)

The use of an applied chromophore to enhance laser energy absorption in tissues is helpful in confining energy penetration to a small volume, while reducing the total laser power required for ablation.[80]

In a study by McNally, Gillings and Dawes in 1999, the topical application of photo-absorbing dye indocyanine green (ICG) to carious lesions in conjunction with laser radiation, allows localized energy deposition. For tissue ablation, this dye has an advantage of binding well to proteins and water and thus it tends to bind to caries rather than to healthy tissue.[80]

The dye exhibits a strong absorption centered at 800 nm and diode laser light at this wavelength is absorbed by caries-dye combination. The risk of thermal damage to surrounding hard and soft tissues is reduced since they absorb near infrared light in this wavelength region poorly.[80]

The results of the study showed that dye-assisted laser ablation technique to be efficient for removal of carious dentin and enamel, with minimal risk of collateral thermal damage. This laser technique is a viable replacement for the dentist's drill producing results with a painless treatment.[80]

Ablation efficiency is directly controlled by cone of ICG dye applied to caries, and concentration of ICG dye applied to caries, and by laser diode power (irradiance). Ablation is selective. No evidence of charring/fissuring was found using SEM. Nor was any evidence of thermal damage, such as discoloration was seen.[80]

The DALA technique was shown to be feasible and it could be developed into a practical method for cavity preparation. The technique offers selective and efficient ablation of carious dentin and enamel as well as pulp sterilization whilst leaving healthy tissue intact.[80]

e. Er, Cr:YSGG Laser Ablation

Erbium, chromium: Yttrium scandium gallium garnet laser was approved for ablation of hard as well as soft tissues by FDA in 1998. BIOLASE has introduced Water Lase system based on Er, Cr:YSGG laser which uses hydrokinetic technology which involves removal of tissues with YSGG laser energized water droplets (Fig. 6.41). Hydrokinetic energy is produced by combining a spray of atomized water with laser energy.[14]

It precisely removes a wide range of human tissue including tooth enamel and soft tissue with no heat and no pain. The wavelength used is 2780 nm at a frequency of 20 Hz with maximum pulse energy of 300 mJ and a maximum power of 6W.[14]

Some of the other applications include:[14]
- Removal of caries
- Root canal cleaning and shaping
- Gingivectomy/frenectomy
- Contouring

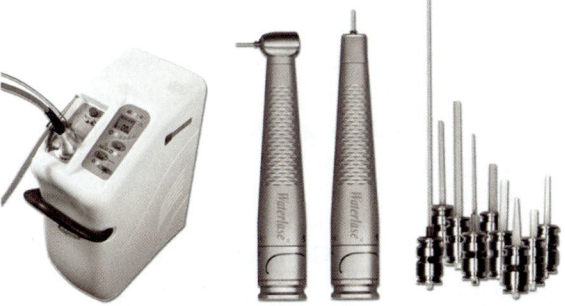

Fig. 6.41: Water-Lase system, handpiece, and tips

Table 6.1: Comparison of benefits of laser over rotary cutting instruments (burs) for cavity preparation

Procedure	Use of burs	Use of lasers
Enamel/dentin cutting	Yes	Yes
Removal of caries selectively	No	Yes
Temperature rise	> 15 degrees	< 5 degrees
Iatrogenic damage	Greater	Lesser
Noise	> 120 dB	< 120 dB
Bactericidal action	No	Surface decontamination
Mode	Contact with tissue mandatory	Non-contact
Pain response	High	Less/none

- Crown lengthening
- Bone ablation
- Apicectomy and
- Periodontal flap surgeries.

f. Diode Laser Ablation

The diode laser is used in the range of 980 nm wavelength which is the second harmonic of the vibrational absorption of 2.94 m erbium wavelength.[14]

A wide variety of esthetic surgical procurers, such as frenectomies, coagulation, and peri-implant soft tissue surgeries are done with this laser.[14]

It is non-contact application performed with optical fibers or a handpiece to treat lesions/cut tissue. It effectively coagulates the vascular lesions and has also been seen to reduce inflammation around the soft tissues.[15]

Maximum output power: 15 W (CW as well as pulsed mode). Since soft tissue has a high percentage of water, the laser must be well absorbed by water. Additionally char free coagulation requires good absorption in hemoglobin.[14] A major benefit of this laser is that it cuts and coagulates optically because of its optimal absorption both in water and hemoglobin.[15]

6. Laser Curing of Composite Resins

Since the early 1980s, use of Argon laser for photo-polymerization of composite resin

restorative material started. The interest arisen because the wavelength (488 nm) of light emitted by the argon laser is optimal for initiation of polymerization of composite resins (Fig. 6.42).[97]

Photo-activated composite resin olymerizes when the initiator (camphoroquinone) in the resin is activated by light. Camphorquinone activation is initiated by a hue of blue light that has a wavelength within the range of 400 to 500 nm with a broad peak activity of 480 nm.[97] Unlike, a VLC unit, the argon laser does not employ the use of filters. Instead, it generates one wavelength of blue light (i.e. monochromaticity) having a band width of only 40–45 nm. In addition, the brightness of light can be set for optimum efficiency unique

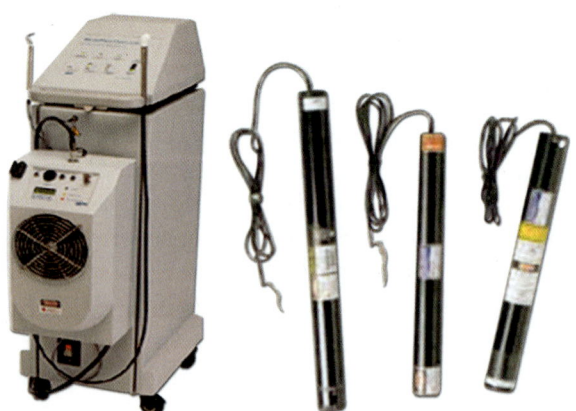

Fig. 6.42: Argon laser curing unit and different laser heads

for each brand.[97] Argon laser emits a collimated (narrow, focused, non-divergent) beam focusing on a specific target, resulting in a more consistent power density over distance.[97]

Advantages[97]

1. The thoroughness and depth of composite resin polymerization are greater with this laser than they are VLC less in polymerized monomer is found in resins cured by argon laser compared to those cured with VLC units.
2. Curing with laser enhances compressive strength, diametral tensile strength, traverse flexural strength and flexural modulus.
3. Wear resistance is equivalent when using either method of polymerization, but argon laser polymerization had demons-trated the potential to improve shear bond strength in both enamel and dentin.
4. Furthermore, laser required less time to achieve equivalent or greater polymeri-zation of restorative material. Argon laser needs only one-fourth of exposure time: 10 seconds for 2 mm depth of cure compared to 40 seconds.

Disadvantages[97]

1. Argon laser curing units are still fairly cumbersome and occupy considerably more space than the conventional VLC units.
2. The laser can generate a substantial amount of heat, cooling fans tends to be noisy and there is a 30 second time lag between turning the units on and actual light emissions.
3. Cost of the argon laser curing unit is a deterrent to its acquisition.
4. Short wavelength light is more energetic than long wavelength light. The argon laser beam is in short wavelength blue light spectrum, which has the highest energy photons of any wavelength of visible light. Its energy level is only slightly less than that of UV light which has a well-documented history of posing a biohazard.
5. There are conflicting reports about the marginal seal obtained with argon laser curing. Increased shrinkage and brit-tleness of some small particle resins has been reported when they have been cured with laser. Pulsed argon laser curing may be the solution for shrinkage problem. Pulsing or periodic interruption of laser beam can be precisely controlled in nanoseconds.

Clinical Significance

As dental technology continue to evolve, new methods of performing certain dental procedures will continue to replace once thought as a pinnacle. The "Argon Laser" may be one such example.[5]

The reduction in polymerization times proved by the argon laser may prove beneficial in reducing chairside time and achieving patient satisfaction. It could be helpful in situations where maintenance of dry field for any length of time is difficult. The increased penetration depth of the argon laser may make possible to cure thicker increments satisfactorily or to cure through thicker sections of tooth.[5]

These advantages make the argon laser an important tool when placing restorations that are complicated or in hard-to-reach areas. On the other hand, narrow focused beam of the laser may make angulations of headpiece more critical in areas of compromised access.[5] The argon laser can also be used to initiate polymerization in any of currently used light activated restorative materials. In addition to restorative composite resins, this family includes bases, liners, pit and fissure sealants and impression materials. Therefore, the argon laser may prove to be quite versatile clinically.[5]

LASER APPLICATIONS IN DENTAL LABORATORY

Applications of laser in dental laboratory includes:
1. Digital laser interferometry.
2. Laser holographic imaging
3. Laser scanning of dental casts
4. Laser fusion of dental casting alloys.

1. Digital laser interferometry: The newest method of measuring polymerization shrinkage of composite materials is digital laser interferometry.[45]

Digital laser interferometry is a procedure based on recording a sequence of interference pattern by using an optoelectronic interferometer. Interferograms are created by superimposing two or more wave fronts of coherent light.[7] To record the two-dimensional fringe patterns of interference of laser beams, a charge-coupled device (CCD) camera is used.[6] And, to process the recorded patterns, a computer program was used. Fringe distribution shows the phase relationship between 2 laser beams. Usually, one beam is called *reference beam* and the other is called *object beam*. Keeping the reference beam constant, a change in fringe distribution of the sequence indicates a deformation of object beam.[6]

The experimental apparatus consists of a low-power He–Ne laser, an interferometer and a computer data acquisition system. In principle, interferometry can be used to detect displacements as small as μ/20 (where μ is the wavelength of He–Ne laser, i.e. 632.8 nm).[45]

Interferometry offers an alternative method to shrinkage measurements that promises improved accuracy and precision.[6] Quality data can be collected over and at a high acquisition rates, permitting the study of primarily fast curing reactions. Linear displacements can be symmetrically measured. The process of extracting the linear shrinkage data from the interferograms is simple in comparison to the dilatometric and strain-gauge/transducer methods, where considerable temperature corrections and gypsum calibration procedures are required to achieve high accuracy and precision.[6]

2. Laser holographic imaging: It is a well-established method for storing topographic information, such as crown preparations, occlusal tables and facial forms. Two laser beams are used which allows more complex surface detail to be mapped using interferometry, while conventional diffraction gratings and interference patterns are used to generate holograms and contour profiles.[70]

3. Laser scanning of dental casts: Laser scanning of dental casts is linked to computerized milling equipment for fabrication of restorations from porcelain (ceramic) and other materials, e.g. CAD-CAM system.[70]

4. Laser fusion of dental casting alloys: Beginning with their inception in 1960s, lasers have been used in welding of metals, laser light is a coherent light, which makes it possible to focus the energy on a fixed position and under certain conditions to weld (or fuse) the pieces being joined without physical contact. Because the weld area is soft and small, the heat input occur for a very short time, thus a weld can be made close to glass or organic materials, such as ceramics or plastic materials.[75]

It offers a method which allows welding on the master cast or in the transfer record from the intraoral relationship. A more appropriate term is 'Laser fusion' which is now currently used.[75]

Laser fusion of gold alloys and type III non-precious alloys is commonly practiced.

The major advantages of laser fusion are:[38]

1. Laser melting and solidification did not alter the properties of welded alloy.
2. Hardness was comparable to that of conventional casting methods.
3. Ability to age harden was not changed.
4. Strength of laser-welded joints is more uniform than soldered connections of same alloy.
5. Did not exhibit significant undesirable characteristics.
6. Rapid and convenient method.
7. Strength is comparable to the annealed strength of alloys fused together.

7

Low-Level Laser Therapy (LLLT)

INTRODUCTION

While the lasers already mentioned can be labeled *"High-level lasers"*, there is a less known type of lasers called *"Low-level lasers"*. These lasers are generally smaller, less expensive and operate in the milliwatt range, 1–500 milliwatts. The therapy performed with such lasers is often called "Low-level laser therapy" (LLLT) and the lasers are called "therapeutic lasers". Several other names have been given to these lasers, such as "soft laser" and "low intensity level laser" whereas the therapy has been referred to as "biostimulation" and "biomodulation". The latter term is more appropriate, since the therapy cannot only stimulate, but also suppress biological processes. Other terms often used for these lasers are 'cold lasers' and 'quantum healing lasers'.

Low-level laser therapy has been utilized in humans since early 1970s. Initially, this form of energy delivery was used to support wound healing (*therapeutic laser treatment*) but now it

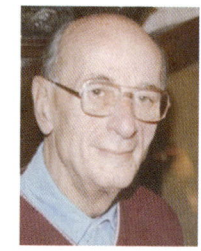

Professor Andre Mester

Discovered the benefits of low-powered laser light in 1964

is also used to accelerate wound healing, minimize pain and reduce inflammatory responses. [142] Low-level lasers are commonly employed in LLLT because of their lower costs and their simplicity of use. [13]

The triage of dental treatment can be summarized as the control/eradication of disease, control/relief of pain and restoration of form/function. The interrelationship of any stimulus with injury, cellular response and pain can be the product of nature and the potency of stimulus and the ability of the tissue to respond (Fig. 7.1).

Low-level laser therapy involves the use of visible red and near-infrared light with tissue in order to stimulate and improve healing as well as reduce pain.

The first low-level laser introduced was **helium–neon (He–Ne),** a gas emitting laser with a wavelength in the visible light spectrum ($\lambda = 632.8$ nm) and a low power output of 1 to 5 mW in mid to late 1970s by Senda et al.[105] However, the wavelength produced by He–Ne laser was highly absorbed by soft tissues, its penetration was limited. So, newer diode/semiconductor lasers were developed that could penetrate soft tissues without damaging them.[13]

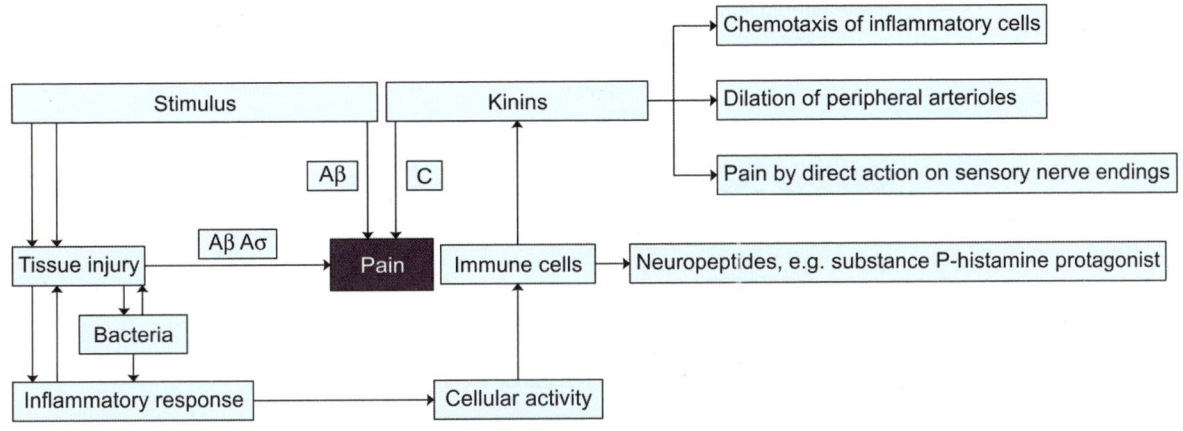

Fig. 7.1: Interrelationship between response, stimulus and pain

The most popular was **gallium–arsenide (GaAs)** with a wavelength of 904 nm and a power output of 1–4 mW. **The GaAlAs (gallium–aluminium–arsenide) laser** was developed in 1980 which emit in the near-infrared spectrum (780 nm, 830 nm and 900 nm) with a power output of 10–30 mW.[13] The first use of GaAlAs laser was reported by Matsumoto et al in combination with chemical agents, such as stannous fluoride which enhanced its effectiveness by more than 20%.[105]

The **InGaAlP (indium-gallium-aluminum phosphide) laser** was developed in mid 1990s, which emit wavelengths in the red spectrum of visible light (630 to 700 nm) with a power output of 25 to 50 mW. They offer an alternative to He–Ne laser for surface wound healing.

Combination probes of two laser wavelengths or more laser diodes with LEDs of various wavelengths may be made as 'cluster probes'. [60]

Contact mode is needed for all applications, when contacting dental structures (enamel, dentin) some fluid might be needed to ensure full contact between the probe and surface to minimize loss of energy.[60]

MECHANISM OF LLLT

The principle of using LLLT is to supply direct biostimulative light energy to the body's cells (Figs 7.2 and 7.3). Cellular photoreceptors (e.g. cytochromophores) can absorb low-level laser light and pass it on to mitochondria which promptly produces the cell fuel: **ATP**.[60]

The most recognized theory to explain the effects and mechanisms of LLLT is the **photochemical theory**. According to this theory, light is absorbed by certain molecules, followed by a cascade of biologic events suggested photoreceptors are endogenous porphyrins and molecules in the respiratory chain, such as cytochrome C-oxidase, leading to increased ATP production.[60]

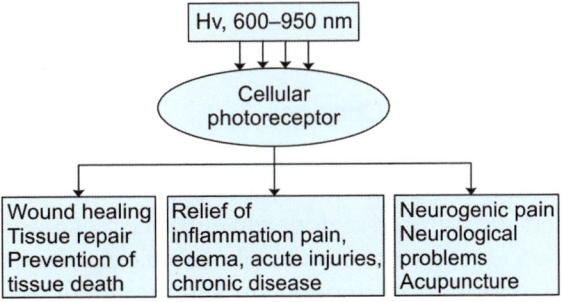

Fig. 7.2: Principle of low-level laser therapy

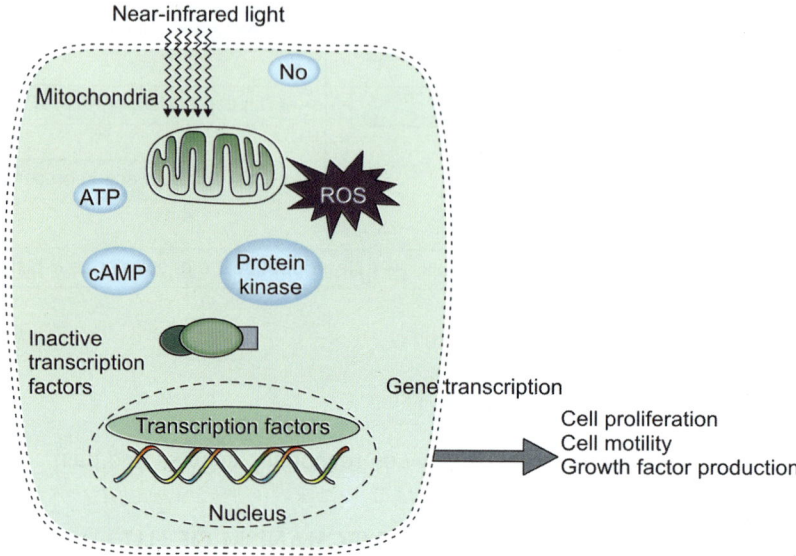

Fig. 7.3: Mechanism of LLLT which takes place inside a cell

How does it Work?

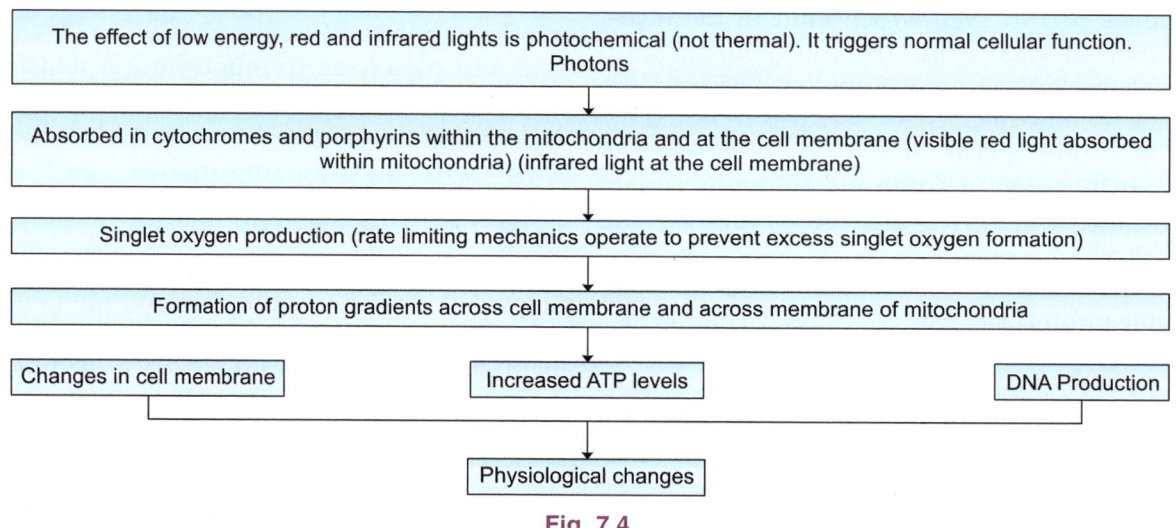

Fig. 7.4

Physiological Changes

Thus, it is possible to conclude that irradiation with monochromatic visible light in the blue, red and infrared regions can enhance metabolic processes in the cell. The photobiologic effects of stimulation depend on the wavelengths, dose and intensity of the light.[60]

LLLT Unit (Fig. 7.5)

Low level laser units are much smaller, often self-contained hand-held devices which are either battery driven or charge via a pod in a bench top master unit. Since an increased temperature of a diode laser device during operation reduces the output power (and to a

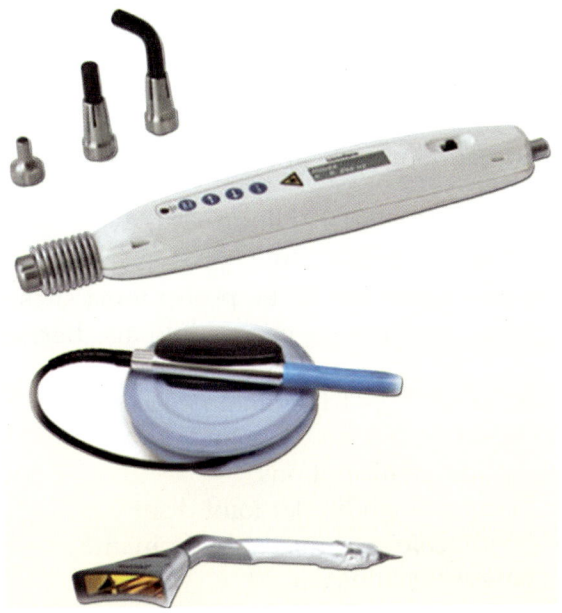

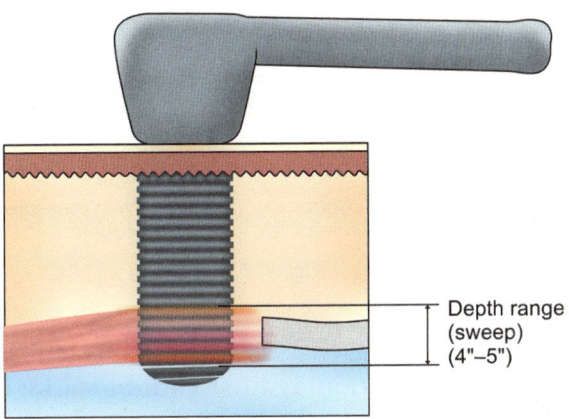

Depth range
(sweep)
(4"–5")

Fig. 7.6

Fig. 7.5: Low-level laser devices with different tips

lesser extent also lengthens the wavelength), it is critical that the temperature or output of the laser diode is monitored so that control circuitry can make the necessary adjustments to maintain a constant output. This is usually accomplished using an internal photo-transistor which is fitted within the package of the laser device. With an adequate heat sink and cooling system (with Peltier cooling for higher powered devices), the potential negative effect of temperature on laser output at the level of the treatment beam can virtually be eliminated.

Power outputs are typically in the order of 10–50 mW, when measured at the level of the diode laser itself. It is important to note that the final useable output (from the handpiece) will be less because of losses in the internal optical path or in the delivery system.

The beam profile from a typical diode laser is rectangular, with a high divergence on the long axis (20 degrees from the center axis), and a low divergence on the short axis (2 degrees).

This gives a highly divergent oval or 'sweep' profile. Diode lasers may have integrated optics which produce collimated and focused light beams. To obtain a more useful beam, a series of lenses or a self-focusing graded index fiber can be used in front of the device to either deliver the treatment beam itself or to direct the laser output into a small diameter flexible optical fibre or a solid light guide (similar to the light tip on a curing light).

Whatever the delivery system used, it is important that the components which come into direct contact with patients are able to be protected adequately with a laser-transmissive disposable barrier, can be autoclaved, or are disposable. Similarly, it should be possible for the clinician to activate the laser into treatment mode without breaching asepsis. Some units employ footswitches or light-operated switches to allow hands-free operation. Laser units used for LLLT are generally classified as Class III or Class IIIb in terms of the optical hazards which they pose to staff and patients. Because a low power treatment beam can be focused by the eye to give a high power density on the retina, the optical hazard is sufficiently great that laser safety standards mandate the wearing of appropriate pro-tective glasses by patients and clinicians

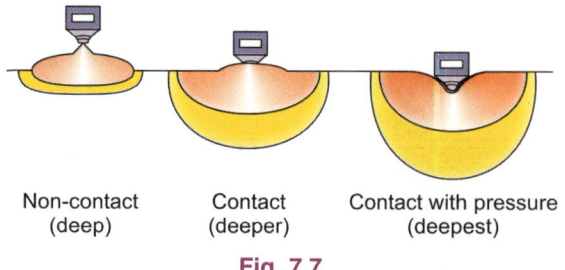

| Non-contact (deep) | Contact (deeper) | Contact with pressure (deepest) |

Fig. 7.7

during treatment. Glasses are available which provide protection against common LLLT wavelengths in both the visible and near infrared spectrum.

Dosimetry

The dosimetry of low level laser light is crucial to the infrasurgical effects of wavelengths used. This is based on Arndt-Schultz law. This is summarized as "small doses stimulate living systems, medium doses impede and large doses destroy". The **energy** used is indicated in *joule (J)*, which is the number of milliwatts × the number of seconds of irradiation. Thus, 50 mW × 60 seconds produces energy of 3000 millijoules, equals 3 J. Suitable therapeutic energies range from 1–10 J per point. The **dose** is expressed in J/cm^2. To calculate the dose, the irradiated area must be known. 1 J over an area of 1 cm^2 = 1 J/cm^2. 1 J over an area of 0.1 cm^2 = 10 J/cm^2. There is generally no heat sensation or tissue heating involved in this therapy. The incident fluence increasing through a range of infra-ablative values gave rise to cellular effects as follows:

a. < 60 mJ/cm^2 : Zero bioactivation
b. 120–240 mJ/cm^2 : Biostimulation
c. 240–300 mJ/cm^2 : Zero bioactivation
d. 300–600 mJ/cm^2 : Bioinhibition

In clinical practice, low level laser therapy, effective through stimulatory rather than ablative mechanisms delivers fluences of 2–10 mJ/cm^2 depending on the target tissues as follows:

- Oral epithelium and gingival tissue: 2–3 J/cm^2
- Transosseous irradiation (periapical tissue): 2–4 mJ/cm^2
- Extraoral muscle groups/TMJ: 6–10 J/cm^2

Clinical Applications in Dentistry (Fig. 7.8)

- Dentin hypersensitivity
- Post-extraction socket/post-trauma sites
- Viral infections—herpes labialis, herpes simplex
- Neuropathy—trigeminal neuralgia, paresthesia
- Aphthous ulcerations
- Temporomandibular joint disorders
- Postoncology—mucositis, dermatitis, post-surgery healing

How does Low-Level Laser Therapy (LLLT) Benefit Patients? [87]

- Relieves acute and chronic pains
- Increases the speed, quality and tensile strength of tissue repair
- Increases blood supply
- Stimulates the immune system
- Stimulates nerve function
- Develops collagen and muscle tissue
- Helps generate new and healthy cells and tissue
- Promotes faster wound healing and clot formation
- Reduces inflammation

Is Low-Level Laser Therapy more Effective than High Energy Irradiation?

Studies have shown that LLLT produces a biological effect in increasing the potential of action of pulp tissue and low-energy wavelengths produced are safer to the pulp because they stimulate circulation and cellular activity. Since low-level irradiation is mostly related to bio-stimulation and analgesia, such

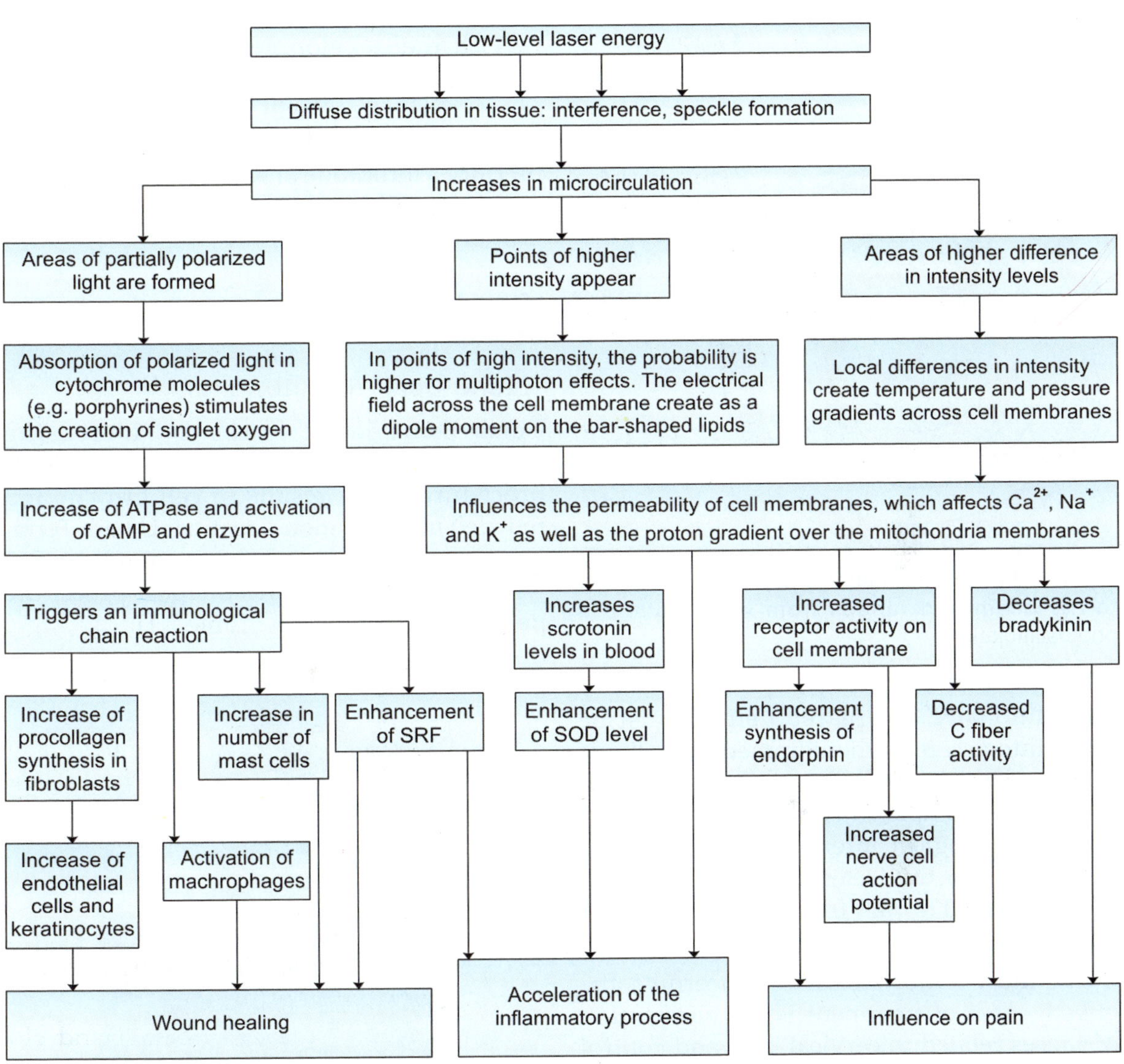

Low-level laser energy

Diffuse distribution in tissue: interference, speckle formation

Increases in microcirculation

Areas of partially polarized light are formed

Points of higher intensity appear

Areas of higher difference in intensity levels

Absorption of polarized light in cytochrome molecules (e.g. porphyrines) stimulates the creation of singlet oxygen

In points of high intensity, the probability is higher for multiphoton effects. The electrical field across the cell membrane create as a dipole moment on the bar-shaped lipids

Local differences in intensity create temperature and pressure gradients across cell membranes

Increase of ATPase and activation of cAMP and enzymes

Influences the permeability of cell membranes, which affects Ca^{2+}, Na^{+} and K^{+} as well as the proton gradient over the mitochondria membranes

Triggers an immunological chain reaction

Increases scrotonin levels in blood

Increased receptor activity on cell membrane

Decreases bradykinin

Increase of procollagen synthesis in fibroblasts

Increase in number of mast cells

Enhancement of SRF

Enhancement of SOD level

Enhancement synthesis of endorphin

Decreased C fiber activity

Increase of endothelial cells and keratinocytes

Activation of machrophages

Increased nerve cell action potential

Wound healing

Acceleration of the inflammatory process

Influence on pain

Fig. 7.8: The diagram represents the process initiated by the energy emitted from a low-level laser and the physical impact of that laser as well as the potential effects resulting from the application from laser energy

effects are temporary. The role of 'soft laser' as a therapeutic tool is thus a contentious issue (Fig. 7.9).[84]

HLLT, on the other hand, is also a better option for management of hypersensitive teeth, if appropriate parameters are maintained to prevent irreversible damage to the pulp. Since, an increased number of tubules per unit area are observed in sensitive dentin and tubule diameters are twice as wide when compared with non-sensitive teeth, lasers act by blocking dentinal tubules are more likely to provide long-term pain relief. HLLT produces rapid and lasting pain relief.[84]

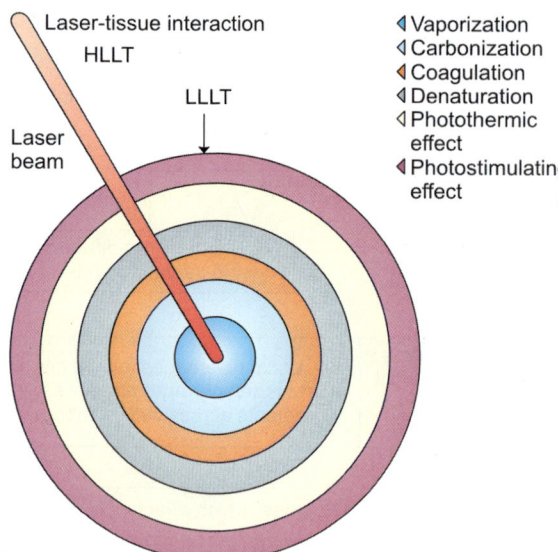

Laser-tissue interaction
HLLT
LLLT
Laser beam

◁ Vaporization
◁ Carbonization
◁ Coagulation
◁ Denaturation
◁ Photothermic effect
◁ Photostimulating effect

Fig. 7.9: Effect of laser energy depends on proximity to the beam and ranges from vaporization to photostimulation

Additionally, the placebo effect must be taken into account where immediate relief is obtained with laser therapy. This effect consists of a complex mixture of physiological and psychological interactions, depending considerably on the doctor–patient relationship. This is thought to vary from 20–60% in dentin hypersensitivity clinical trials.[84]

The most important issue concerning the effectiveness of treatment is the elimination of causes related to cervical pain and control of primary causes of dental erosion and dentin exposure. Modification of dietary habits is essential since dietary acids contribute to dentinal hypersensitivity and influence its treatment. Therefore, patients should be counseled about the quantity and frequency of acid intake and cautioned against brushing too soon after acid ingestion. Elimination of gastric regurgitation problems and establishment of proper oral hygiene techniques are important as well to promote therapy.[84]

With the development of thinner, more flexible and durable laser fibers, laser application in dentistry will increase. Ideally, the laser of the future will have the ability to produce a multitude of wavelengths and pulse widths, each specific to a particular application.[60]

LOW-LEVEL LASER DEVICES AVAILABLE

1. Terra-Dent (Fig. 7.10)

Terra-Dent laser works by increasing circulation in the micro cells affected by dental procedures. This results in cell growth and reduced inflammation. Treatments with Terra-Dent may also help to prevent complications, which often arise during the post-procedure period due to infection (Table 7.1).

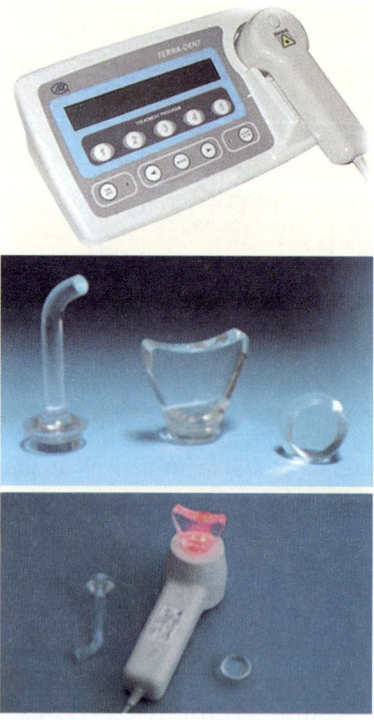

Fig. 7.10: Terra-Dent laser with dental probes or accessories

Mechanism behind Terra-Dent

Terra-Dent laser involves the use of **multi radiance technology** (MRT). MRT was engineered to allow one laser emitter device to produce the power and range of spectrum from superficial to the deepest bone and hard tissue. It combines superficial 660 nm red light with medium penetrating 875 nm infrared, and deep penetrating 905 nm super-pulsed infrared laser, plus magnetic induction for enhancing microcirculation. Multi-radiance technology (MRT) uses multiple therapeutic radiances (four healing energies) working together for the absolute best biologic cellular response from skin to bones and everything in between. MRT has a unique combination of four radiances, which is perfect for optimal pain relief and quickened healing.

The Core Concepts Behind Multi-Radiance Technology

1. **Super pulsed laser** (905 nm): A high power of impulse light at a billionth of a second. This high power during each pulse drives the light to the target tissue, up to a depth of 10–13 cm (4–5 inches). The Terra-Dent's high-peak power of up to 25,000 mW generates a high photon density, delivering the dense concentration of photons for healing which provides extraordinarily deep tissue saturation. Super-pulsed laser can influence pain reduction, improves the circulation at the tips of the blood vessels and improves ATP production which facilitates cellular metabolism (Fig. 7.11).

2. **Pulsed broad band infrared emitting diodes** (875 nm) is useful at higher tissue depths than the laser but provide a wider spectrum-compared to laser radiation by slightly heating the upper tissue.

3. **Pulsed red light** (660 nm) penetrates shallower tissue depth and has anti-inflammatory benefits.

4. **Static magnetic field** keeps ionized molecules of tissue in a dissociated stage, enhancing the energy potential at the molecular and cellular levels.

Working together, these multiple radiances induce biology conducive to healing and pain relief. When used at preset frequencies, you can control the depth of the therapeutic energy from the surface up to 13 cm (5 inches) deep.

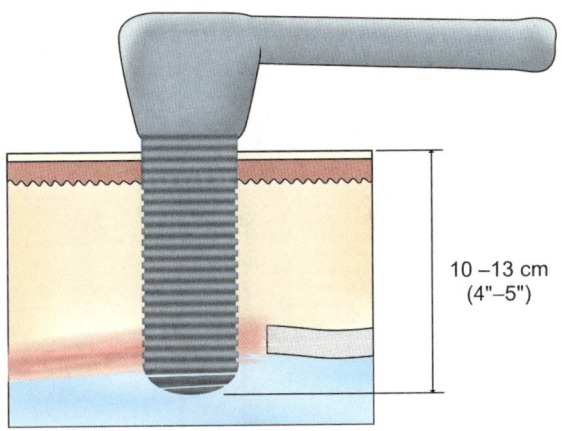

10 –13 cm
(4"–5")

Fig. 7.11: Super pulsing allows for deeper penetration than a laser of the same wavelength that is not super-pulsed but has the same average output power. This is because ultimately short pulses allow for quick absorption at the cellular level. And the period between pulses promotes a better environment for enhanced cell communication, leading to an optimum pain relief and accelerated healing

Benefits
- Reduces pain by increase of serotonin level
- Increases circulation in tiny cells
- Stimulates fibroblasts and osteoblasts
- Effective for nerve injuries and TMJ
- Reduces swelling and hypersensitivity
- Increases healing of soft tissue and bone
- Increases release of B-endorphins

2. Dr. M Laser Tooth Brush

It is the world's first semiconductor medical toothbrush that utilizes low level laser therapy. This toothbrush treats dentin

Program	1	2	3	4	5
Treatment	Soft tissue healing	Specific treatment programs	Implants and bone regenerate	Post-surgical pain (acute)	Chronic pain
Pulse frequency	1000 Hz/sec	5–100 variation Hz/sec	250–1000 variation Hz/sec	50 Hz/sec	5–50 variation Hz/sec
Program duration	5 minutes	5 minutes	5 minutes	5 minutes	4 minutes

Table 7.1: Terra-Dent laser programs

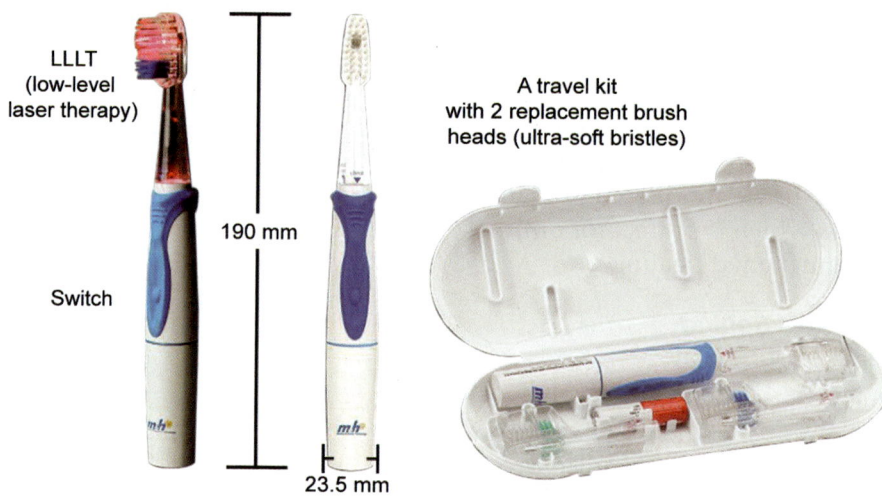

Fig. 7.12: Laser tooth brush kit

hypersensitivity and alleviates tooth ache. The laser beam is emitted only when main body is hold and toothbrush sensor is contacted after mode switch is pressed.

All the functions in Dr. M toothbrush is controlled by a built-in micro-computer (micom). Its laser technology also prevents dental caries thus allowing maintenance oral hygiene and healthy oral cavity (Fig. 7.12).

Conclusion

Low level laser therapy has been found to accelerate wound healing and reduce pain, possibly by stimulating oxidative phosphory-lation in mitochondria and modulating inflammatory responses. By influencing the biological function of a variety of cell types, it is able to exert a range of several beneficial effects upon inflammation and healing.

Future trials of new LLLT applications in dentistry should make use of standardized, validated outcomes, and should explore how the effectiveness of the LLLT protocol used may be influenced by wavelength, treatment duration, dosage, and the site of application.

8

Lasers in Endodontics

After initial experiments with the ruby laser, clinicians began using other lasers, such as argon (Ar), carbon dioxide (CO_2), Nd:YAG and Er:YAG lasers.[141]

The first laser used in endodontics was reported by Weichman and Johnson (1971) who attempted to seal the apical foramen in vitro by means of high power infrared (CO_2) laser. Although this goal was not achieved, sufficient relevant and interesting data were obtained to encourage further study.[141]

The rapid development of laser technology, as well as better understanding of their interaction with biological tissues, has widened the spectrum of possible applications of lasers in endodontics.[141]

The development of new delivery systems, including thin and flexible fibers as well as new endodontic tips, has made it possible to apply this technology to various endodontic procedures, such as:

- Pulpal diagnosis
- Pulp capping/pulpotomy
- Cleaning and disinfecting of root-canal system.
- Obturation of root-canal system
- Endodontic re-treatment, and
- Apical surgery

A. ENDODONTIC DIAGNOSIS

1. Assessment of Pulpal Blood Flow by Laser Doppler Flowmetry

Laser Doppler flowmetry (LDF) was first introduced in 1970s by Morikawa et al to assess blood flow in microvascular systems, e.g. in retina, gut mesentery, renal cortex and skin (Riva et al, 1972).[141]

Use: He–Ne and GaAlAs semiconductor diode lasers at a low power of 1 or 2 mW are used in laser Doppler flowmetry. The wavelength of the He–Ne laser is 632.8 nm and that of the semiconductor diode laser, 780 to 820 nm. To prevent laser beams from reflecting off of the surrounding gingival, the measurement of the laser beams reflected from the dental pulp should be carried out under the rubber dam.[118]

The **principle** in the diagnosis of pulp vitality by laser Doppler flowmetry is based on the changes in red blood cell flux in the pulp tissue. It is difficult to obtain the laser reflection from some teeth. The anterior teeth, in which the enamel and dentin are thin, generally do not present a problem. In the molar teeth, the enamel and dentin are thicker. The advantage of this diagnostic method is that it allows painless diagnosis. The laser Doppler flowmetry method is useful in

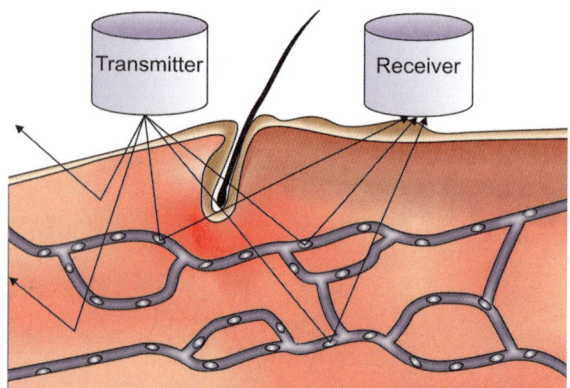

Fig. 8.1: Basic operating principle of laser Doppler flowmetry. A laser beam is directed to an area of tissue. Upon contact with red blood cells in the target tissue, light waves are reflected and scattered, resulting in broadening of the light wave frequency, which is detected and received by a photodetector

detection of pulp vitality of immature or traumatized teeth and for patients who are sensitive to tooth pain (Fig. 8.1).[124]

Odor, Pitt Ford, McDonald (1996) investigated the effect of wavelength and bandwidth on laser Doppler flowmeter signals from vital and root-filled teeth, and to establish their sensitivity and specificity (Table 8.1). There was a highly significant difference between readings from vital and root-filled teeth for the 3.1 kHz/810 nm wavelength combination ($p < 0.003$) and a significant difference for the 3.1 kHz/633 nm wavelength group ($p < 0.02$). The 810 nm wavelength showed good sensitivity but poor specificity at 14.9 and 22.1 kHz bandwidths. The 633 nm wavelength showed good specificity, but poor sensitivity, at 14.9 and 22.1 kHz bandwidths. The 3.1 kHz

bandwidth showed the best sensitivity and specificity for both wavelengths. The 810 nm/ 3.1 kHz combinations offered the greatest sensitivity and specificity as a test to distinguish between root-filled and vital teeth. This combination was best.[124]

Table 8.1 shows laser characteristics used in LDF.[141]

The lasers used for LDF are usually at a low-power level of 1 or 2 mW with no reports of pulp injury. The first study showing that LDF could differentiate b/w vital and non-vital pulps in humans was published in 1986 by Gazelius et al.[141]

One of the first studies to confirm that it was actually blood flow that was being measured in pulp with LDF was by Kim et al in 1990. The initial use of LDF was exclusively for direct soft tissue blood flow measurements, without any interference of hard tissues like enamel or dentin.[118]

Chaiyavej, Yamamoto, et al (2000) investigated the response of intradental A and C fibers during tooth cutting by Er:YAG laser. They concluded that during the tooth cutting, Er:YAG laser was more effective in activating intradental A fibers compared with micromotor and also caused the activation of intradental C fibers.[124]

The effec of irradiation with a gallium–aluminum–arsenide semiconductor laser on responses evoked in trigeminal subnucleus caudal neurons by tooth pulp stimulation was investigated electrophysiologically in Wister rats anesthetized with urethane plus alpha-chloralose by Wakabayashi, Hamba, et al (1993). The study indicated that low power

Table 8.1: Laser characteristics used in LDF			
Lasers	Penetration ability (E and D thickness of 3 mm)	Specificity	Sensitivity
He–Ne (633 nm)	2.11%	Good	Poor
GaAlAs (810–830 nm)	3.91%	Poor	Good

laser irradiation (semiconductor laser: 830 nm, 350 mW, CW, through the tooth structures, for 120s) inhibited the excitation of unmyelinated fibers of the pulp without affecting fine myelinated fibers. Hence the results suggest tsthe depolarization of C fiber afferents (Fig. 8.2).[141]

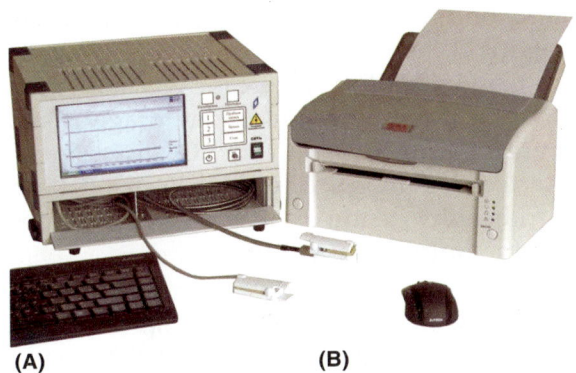

(A)   **(B)**

Fig. 8.2: Laser Doppler instrumentation: (A) Scanning laser Doppler imager, (B) single point fiber optic monitor with fiberoptic probes

Other Applications of LDF [141]

1. To assess pulpal blood blow in primary incisors, prior to pulpotomy or extractions.
2. As a useful adjunct for luxated teeth.
3. To identify "at-risk" teeth early after the trauma.
4. To assess revascularization of traumatized teeth.

Drawbacks of LDF[141]

1. High initial set up cost.
2. Inconsistent readings and assessment over time (to be able to obtain accuracy and consistency, certain critical steps need to be taken. First, because of the sensitivity to movement, it is not possible to hold the probe manually against a crown surface. A stabilizing stent, made out of rubber important material needs to be fabricated individually for each patient. This will not only reduce the artificial movements that might be easily picked up by photodetectors but also ensure that the tooth is always tested on the same part of the crown. Prior to placing the stent, the gingiva should be covered with dark-dental dam or aluminum foil).

3. Not established that LDF provide a reliable indication of changes in red cell flux of pulp tissue under physiological conditions due to problems, such as artifacts; e.g.
   • Indication of changes in red cell flux of gingival tissue
   • Changes in ambient light intensity, and
   • Movement artifacts.

2. Heat Stimulation by Laser Instead of Hot Gutta-percha

The hot gutta-percha method is commonly applied for the differential diagnosis of vital versus non-vital dental pulp. This method has a disadvantage in that pain response cannot always be obtained because of the thick enamel and dentin or the high pain perception threshold of the dental pulp. The laser stimulation method by pulsed Nd:YAG laser was reported to be mild and tolerable compared with the pain induced by the conventional electric pulp tester.[43]

In addition to the pulsed Nd:YAG laser, other lasers may be used to diagnose the difference between vital and non-vital dental pulp in the future. Intracanal laser-softened gutta-percha, ultrafil, and intracanal laser-cured composite resin techniques were compared with respect to the temperature elevation induced on the outer root surface in a study by Matsumoto (1995).[43] The temperature at the root surface of 50 single-rooted teeth was measured using a thermovision camera. Argon laser produced a rise in temperature of +12.9°C (gutta-percha) and +13.3°C (composite resin), respectively.[43]

The CO_2 laser produced +10.3°C and Nd:YAG laser produced the highest temperature elevation of +14.4°C. Low-temperature gutta-percha obturation technique did not produce a measurable temperature change on the external root surfaces. Anil, and Matsumoto (1995), compared the effectiveness of four different techniques used for obturation of single-rooted teeth: lateral condensation, low-temperature gutta-percha (ultrafil), vertical condensation of gutta-percha softened by means of three different laser devices (argon, CO_2, and Nd:YAG), or composite resin photo-polymerized by argon laser.[43] The most extensive dye penetration (4.3 mm) was observed in teeth obturated with composite resin, followed by gutta-perch laser with CO_2 (2.15 mm), and the Nd:YAG laser (3.54 mm).[43]

Gutta-percha softened with argon laser created an apical seal almost identical to that obtained with the lateral condensation and ultrafil techniques (1.50, 1.45, and 1.48 mm of leakage, respectively). These results indicate that the argon laser can be used for gutta-percha softening to produce good apical sealing results. [43]

3. Differential Diagnosis of Pulpitis by Laser Stimulation

Normal pulp and acute pulpitis: When normal pulp is stimulated by the pulsed Nd:YAG laser at 2 W and 20 pulses per second (pps) at a distance of approximately 10 mm from the tooth surface, pain is produced within 20 to 30 seconds and disappears a couple of seconds after the laser stimulation is stopped. In the case of acute pulpitis, the pain is induced immediately after laser application and continues for more than 30 seconds after stopping the laser stimulation.[141]

Acute serous pulpitis and acute suppurative pulpitis: Differential diagnosis of acute serous pulpitis and acute suppurative pulpitis can be obtained by combining the measurement of electric current resistance of caries and the pain duration induced by laser stimulation. If the electric current resistance is greater than 15.0 mW and the patient experiences continuous pain for more than 30 seconds, the diagnosis is acute serous pulpitis. When the value of the resistance is less than 15.0 mW and there is continuous pain for more than 30 seconds, the diagnosis is acute suppurative pulpitis. Carious impedance of less than 15.0 mW indicates that no hard healthy dentin exists between the caries and the pulp chamber.[141]

B. PEDIATRIC ENDODONTICS (Pulp-Capping and Pulpotomy) (Fig. 8.3)

According to American Association of Endodontists (AAE), *pulp capping is a "procedure in which a dental material is applied on an exposed or nearly exposed dental pulp in order to stimulate the formation of irritation dentin in the exposed area."*[25]

COHEN and BURNS defined the treatment as: *"pulp capping is the application of a medicament or dressing to the exposed pulp in an attempt to preserve vitality".* The technological progress in the field of preserving pulpal vitality after accidental, traumatic or caries-related pulpal exposure justifies the efficiency of laser equipment. It improves clinical and biological status of treated pulp tissue, due to its wound conditioning ability through dis-infection, dentinal tubule sealing and hemostatic control.[25]

The types of lasers used in pulp treatment procedures are: CO_2, Nd:YAG, Er:YAG, Er: Cr: YSGG, 980 nm and 810 nm GaAlAs diode laser.[25]

Tuner and Hode considered that laser therapy can be recommended for pulp capping and pulp amputation of deciduous teeth. Laser therapy appears to stimulate odontoblast calcium and collagen production, leading to secondary dentin formation.[25]

According to Gutknecht et al, pulpotomy is a very common technique in pediatric dentistry and CO_2 laser is described very effective for this technique. The major advantage of CO_2 laser in the field of preserving pulp vitality is its thermal effect; it sterilizes and heals the irradiated area, ensures a close contact between the dental pulp and capping agent by reducing inflammation and size of blood clot and may help in preventing bacterial microinfiltration which is the key factor in pulp-capping failure.[25] Apart from these effects, *Holz* concluded that CO_2 laser has the ability to stimulate dentinogenesis process.[25] According to Moritz et al, CO_2 laser is an easy, safe and fast method for hemostasis; disinfection and sealing of exposed pulp tissue, especially, because it is possible to operate CO_2 laser in super-pulsed mode, thus considerably reducing the thermal effect on adjacent tissues.[141]

Nd:YAG lasers are also capable of reducing dentin permeability, thus they are recommended for conditioning the remaining dentin layer by sealing dentinal tubules.[25]

Er:YAG, Er: Cr:YSGG lasers are also used to perform caries removal, coagulation of exposed pulp, pulpotomy or pulpectomy.[56]

The first laser pulpotomy was performed by Shoji et al in 1985; they used CO_2 laser in focused and defocused mode with power levels of 3, 10, 30 and 60 W in dental pulp of dogs.[141] They noticed coagulation necrosis and degeneration of odontoblastic cell layer, without damaging radicular pulp tissue. Moritz et al (1998) reported that CO_2 laser was a valuable aid in direct pulp capping in human patients.[141]

In 2001, Jayewardene et al evaluated the response of accidentally exposed dental pulp in rodents to Er:YAG laser (150 mJ/pulse, 10 pulses of wavelength 2.94) 3 days and 2 weeks after treatment. The laser-treated group showed a higher frequency of dentin bridge formation compared to control group.[141]

When lasers are used in pulp capping to create the biological base for the formation of sterile area, the creation of dentinal bridge and for maintenance of pulp vitality, following may be considered as contributing factors:

1. The sterile area is due to the bactericidal effect of laser, an effect common to all the laser wavelengths. The CO_2 and erbium group of lasers are more superficial in their interaction with tissue than diode and Nd:YAG wavelengths, which penetrate more deeply (up to 500 to 1000 µm) and have greater capacity for scattering.[56] The decontaminating action of laser, more or less superficial, must be completed with immediate sealing of exposed pulp area to avoid recontamination through leakage.[56]

2. The coagulating effect of laser guarantees a dry operating area, with no bleeding and the creation of a zone of necrosis that is more superficial compared to a chemical pulp-capping agent. (Different lasers have different hemostatic/coagulating effects due to differences in absorption by target tissue, i.e. pigment, water or dentin.)[56]

3. In case of a near-exposure of pulpal tissue but without macroscopically evident exposure, a soft, gentle irritation of this limited area with a moderate, controlled thermal effect allows formation of a barrier against bacterial contamination and chemical/mechanical stimuli of pulp tissue.[56]

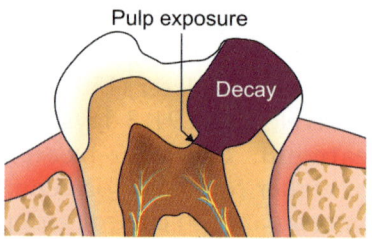

Graphic representation of laser assisted pulp-capping and of formation of dentinal bridge

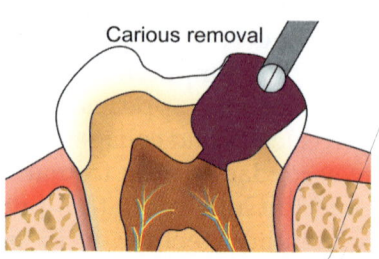

Laser/tissue interaction

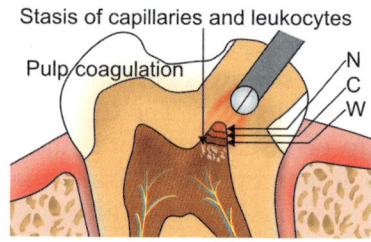

Laser/tissue interaction. N: necrosis area 80°C; C: coagulation area 60°C; W: warming area of reversible damages 35 to 50°C, stasis of capillaries and migration of leukocytes

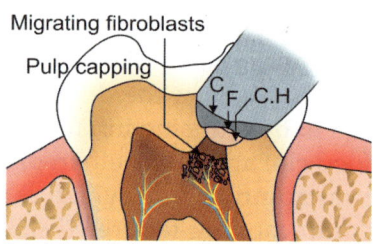

Application of base of calcium hydroxide (CH), immediate filling with flowable composite (F) and microhybrid composite (C): the fibroblasts migrate in the zone under calcium hydroxide, where the dentinal bridge will form

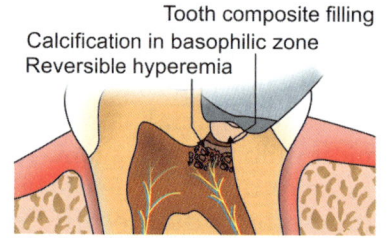

After some weeks, calcification begins

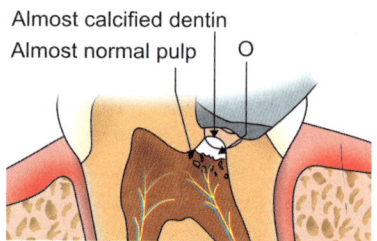

Odontoblasts (O) in the dentinal bridge zone: almost calcified dentin and almost normal pulp

Fig. 8.3: Representation of laser-assisted pulp capping

Conclusion: Laser use in restorative dentistry not only allows improvement in patient approach but also improves the prognosis of treatments, such as pulp capping where maintaining pulpal vitality is a determining factor in clinical success. [56]

C. LASER-ASSISTED ENDODONTICS

The complex root canal anatomy and the limited ability of chemical irrigants to three-dimensionally clean and disinfect the entire endodontic space, the use of lasers was seen as a possible means of adjunctively enhancing the effectiveness of endodontic treatment.

Scientific Basis

The interaction of light on a target follows the rules of optical physics. Light can be reflected, absorbed, diffused, or transmitted. The interaction of laser light with dentin occurs when there is optical affinity between them. This interaction is specific and selective, based on absorption and diffusion. The less affinity, the more light will be transmitted and/or reflected.

The near infrared lasers (from 810 to 1340 nm) have negligible affinity for water and the hydroxyapatite of hard dental tissues and therefore, penetrate to a large extent through dentinal tubules and are absorbed by the bacteria pigments. This allows for a bactericidal effect in deeper dentin layers.

The mid-infrared lasers (2780 and 2940 nm) are primarily absorbed by water (and, to a lesser degree, hydroxyapatite) in the dentinal walls and their bactericidal effect, via photothermal energy, is more superficial. Their affinity for water in dentin also performs a certain amount of ablation of the superficial dentin as a result of the photothermal effect. The carbon dioxide laser (10,600 nm) has a strong affinity for water and especially hydroxyapatite. The inability of this wavelength to utilize a fiberoptic delivery system limits its utility in intracanal applications. In 1999, Kesler et al evaluated the clinical use of a specially designed microprobe (coupled to a CO_2) laser handpiece) within the apical third and reported a level of success comparable to conventional endodontic treatment.

The interaction of different laser wavelengths on different targets (e.g. bacteria, dentin, and irrigants), via absorption or diffusion, generates biological effects responsible for different therapeutic actions that can be summarized as:

- Photothermal effects
- Photochemical effects
- Photothermal effects inducing photo-mechanical and photoacoustic effects.

Effects of Laser Light on Bacteria

At different power levels, all laser wavelengths destroy the cell wall because of their *photothermal effect*. The initial damage takes place in the cell wall via alterations in the osmotic gradient leading to swelling and cellular death. Gram-negative bacteria, due to the structural characteristics of the different cell walls, are more easily destroyed with less energy and less irradiation than gram-positive bacteria.

When erbium laser energy is delivered with very short pulse durations (less than 150 microseconds) in a liquid-filled environment, a shock wave phenomenon (*photomechanical acoustic effect*) can occur. A recent study reported a direct bactericidal effect related to this shock wave-like phenomenon; a bacterial kill of 73% was seen when distilled water was activated by PIPS for 30 seconds in an *ex vivo* infected root canal.

Morphological Effects of Laser Light on the Dentinal Surface

Besides these positive outcomes, the laser thermal effect can generate some damage to the dentin walls. Several studies have investigated the laser-induced morphological effects on root canal walls as collateral sequelae of cleaning and bacterial reduction performed with different lasers. When they are used on dry tissue, both the near-infrared and the mid-infrared lasers produce characteristic thermal effects. Near-infrared lasers cause morphological alterations of the dentinal wall; the smear layer is only partially removed, and the dentinal tubules are primarily closed as a result of melting of the inorganic dentinal structures. Mid-infrared lasers completely vaporize the smear layer, but also produce a superficial thermal phenomenon on the dentin. When used in dry mode in narrow and/or curved canals, these lasers can produce over-enlarging of the coronal section, apical transportation, perforation, and root canal ledging. This is why recent investigations are looking for nonthermal laser bacterial reduction methods, such as photo-activated disinfection (PAD) or LAI.

Effects of Laser Light on Irrigants

Investigations on laser-activated irrigation reported that pulsed erbium lasers can generate a movement of fluids at high speed through a cavitation effect. The expansion (via thermal effect) and successive vapor bubble implosion within irrigant fluids generate a secondary cavitation effect on the intracanal fluids. The pulsed erbium lasers effect on the irrigants within the root canal produced a clean and debrided dentin surface. A particular type of laser activation of irrigants (PIPS) utilizes very low energy (ranging from 50 mJ to 20 mJ) at 10 to 15 Hz delivered with very short pulses (50 microseconds) to generate a more profound shock wave than cavitation. The final effect is similar to the previously described effect with LAI.

Parameters that Influence the Emission of Laser Energy in Endodontics

In addition to the energy and power used, the emission mode of laser light is fundamental for the effects of laser on targets. Diode lasers emit their energy in a continuous-wave (CW) mode. A mechanical interruption of the energy emission is possible (properly called "gated" or "chopped"), allowing for better control of thermal emission and damage. The pulse duration and intervals are measured in milliseconds or microseconds (time on/off).

The Nd:YAG laser and the Erbium laser family emit energy in a "pulsed" mode (also called "free-running pulse"), so that each pulse has a beginning time, increase, and an end time referred to as a Gaussian distribution (Fig. 8.4). Between pulses, the tissue has time to cool somewhat (thermal relaxation time), allowing for better control of thermal effects.

Another important parameter to consider is the length of the pulse (from a few microseconds to milliseconds): shorter pulses (< 150 microseconds) are responsible for higher peak power achievable with less energy and less thermal impact, and longer pulses are responsible for more thermal effects. The tip design also affects the direction and amount of emission of the energy. Traditional laser tips and fibers are end-firing so that no energy is directed laterally. New tips are available today with different designs, tapered and tapered and stripped, so that more energy can be delivered laterally and less frontally.

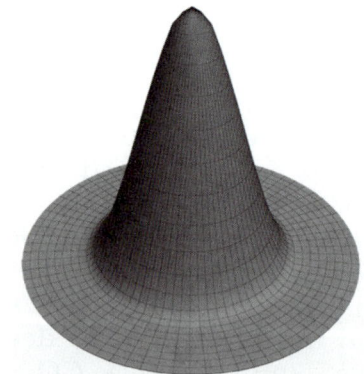

Fig. 8.4: A symmetric bell-shaped curve is the typical shape of the ideal laser beam emitted in TEM00 mode (Gaussian profile)

LASER TECHNIQUES IN ENDODONTICS

Lasers have been used with different techniques in endodontics (Table 8.2):

Table 8.2: Types of laser and techniques used in endodontics

Laser wavelength	Laser technique	Target chromophore	Laser–tissue interaction	Laser effects
Near-infrared	Direct irradiation	Bacteria pigment	Diffusion	Photothermal
Mid-infrared	Direct irradiation	Water content of dentin	Absorption	Photothermal
Visible near-infrared	PAD	Photosensitizers	Absorption	Photochemical
Mid-infrared	LAI	Water content of irrigants	Absorption	Cavitation via photothermal
Mid-infrared	PIPS	Water content of irrigants	Absorption	Cavitation shock wave via photothermal, photomechanical, and photoacoustic

- Traditional laser endodontics (direct laser irradiation) involves the use of end-firing tips or fibers, positioned into the canal, 1 mm shorter than the working length, irradiating while withdrawing the fiber from the canal.

- Photo-activated disinfection (PAD), photodynamic therapy, or light-activated disinfection (LAD) requires the use of different photosensitizers with antimicrobial activity that is selectively activated by different wavelengths.

- Laser-activated irrigation (LAI and PIPS) involves the use of radial-firing tips (which may be tapered, tapered and chemically modified, or tapered and stripped) to improve the lateral emission of photons to activate the irrigants.

TRADITIONAL LASER ENDODONTICS

Bacterial Reduction with Near-Infrared Lasers (Direct Irradiation)

Laser-assisted canal bacterial reduction performed with the near-infrared laser requires the canals to be prepared in the traditional way; the apical preparation is performed with ISO 30/40 files, depending on the laser fiber diameter used. The irradiation is performed at the end of the traditional endodontic treatment, as a final procedure to reduce bacteria in the endodontic system before obturation. A flexible optical fiber of 200–300 micron diameter is placed 1 mm from the apex and withdrawn coronally with different techniques, such as a vertical or helical movement (at 1 or 2 mm/sec according to different procedures).

The Nd:YAG (1064 nm) laser demonstrated a bacterial reduction of three log steps at 1 mm, while in other studies an 810 nm CW diode laser with an output power of 0.6 W achieved a mean bacterial reduction of 74% in a 500 micron slice of dentin and a 980 nm CW diode laser achieved a maximum bacterial reduction of 66% at 2.3 W and 86% at 2.8 W in a 500 micron slice of dentin. These differences in penetration are due to specific optical characteristics of these wavelengths and specific modality of energy emission. The diffusion capacity, which is not uniform, allows the light to reach and destroy bacteria by penetrating via thermal effect.

Many other microbiological studies have confirmed the strong bactericidal action of the diode and Nd:YAG lasers with reduction up to 100% of the bacterial load in the principal canal, but also many studies reported undesirable thermal morphological effects related to the contact of the fiber on the dentinal walls during the withdrawing movement.

Bacterial Reduction with Mid-Infrared Lasers

Given the low efficacy in canal preparation and shaping with the erbium lasers, the use of traditional techniques for canal preparation is required. Canals need to be prepared at the apex with ISO 30/40 instruments. The final passage with the laser is possible through the use of long, thin tips (200 and 320 microns) available from various erbium laser manufacturers, allowing for easier approach to the working length (1 mm from the apex). In this methodology, the traditional technique is to use a helical movement when withdrawing the tip (over a 5–10 sec interval), repeating 3–4 times depending on the procedure. Traditionally these techniques are performed in dry canals and without any irrigation. Moritz et al obtained an almost total eradication of 99.64% of bacteria at 1.5 W, however, these systems did not have a bactericidal effect in penetration depth in the lateral canals.

Stabholz recently reported the development of a new endodontic tip to be used with an Er:YAG laser system.[40] The beam of Er:YAG

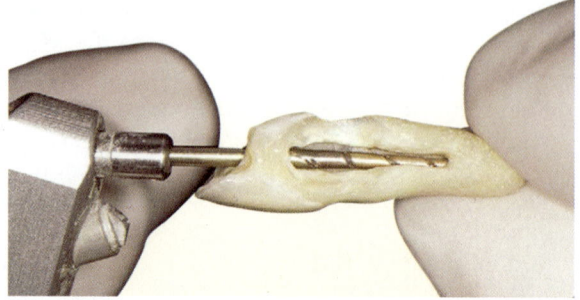

Fig. 8.6: Prototype of RC Lase Side Firing Spiral Tip is shown in root canal of extracted maxillary canine

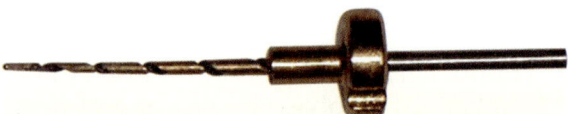

Fig. 8.7: RC Lase Side Firing Spiral Tip

laser is delivered through a hollow tube, with an endodontic tip that allows lateral emission of irradiation, rather than direct emission through a single opening at its far end. This new endodontic tip was designed to fit the shape and volume of root canals. The tip is sealed at its far end, preventing the transmission of irradiation to and through apical foramen of the tooth. These flexible tips come in 275 and 415 micron diameters and 17, 21 and 25 mm lengths (Figs 8.6 to 8.8).

A new area of research has investigated the capacity of the Er:YAG laser for the removal

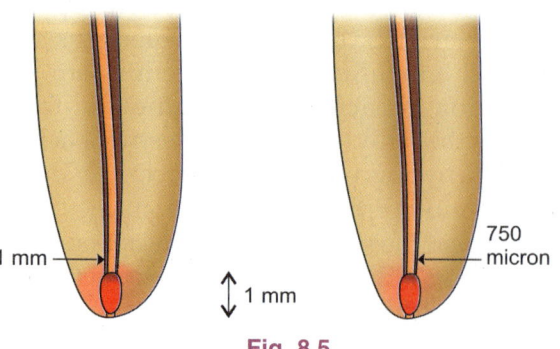

1 mm

750 micron

1 mm

Fig. 8.5

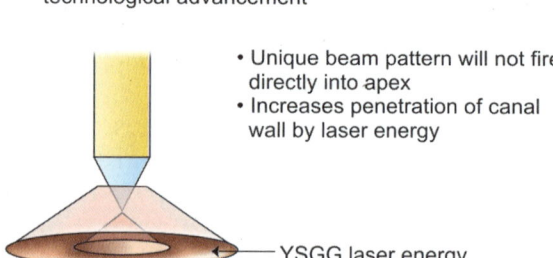

YSGG laser radial firing tips—a technological advancement

• Unique beam pattern will not fire directly into apex
• Increases penetration of canal wall by laser energy

YSGG laser energy

Fig. 8.8: Radiation pattern of radial firing tips

of bacterial biofilm from the apical third and a recent *in vitro* study has further validated the capacity of the Er:YAG laser to remove endodontic biofilm from numerous bacterial species (*Actinomyces naeslundii, Enterococcus faecalis, Propionibacterium acnes, Fusobacterium nucleatum, Porphyromonas gingivalis*, and *Prevotella nigrescens*), with considerable reduction of bacterial cells and disintegration of biofilm. The exception to this was the biofilm formed by *Lactobacillus casei.*

Erbium lasers with "end-firing" tips, with frontal emission at the end of the tip, have little lateral penetration of the dentinal wall, so a radial-emitting tip was proposed in 2007 for the Er,Cr:YSGG laser (Fig. 8.9). Gordon et al have studied the antimicrobial effects and Schoop et al the morphological and bactericidal effects of this laser system (Figs 8.10 and 8.11).

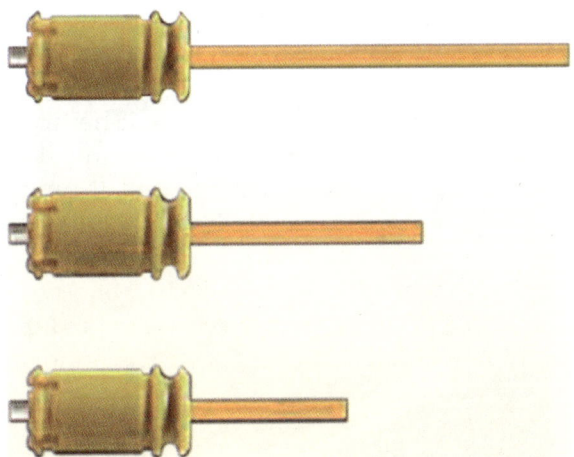

Fig. 8.9: Er, Cr:YSGG laser tips to create endodontic access openings

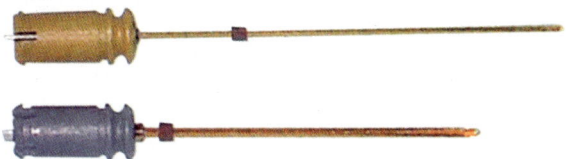

Fig. 8.10: Tips to instrument canals in anterior teeth

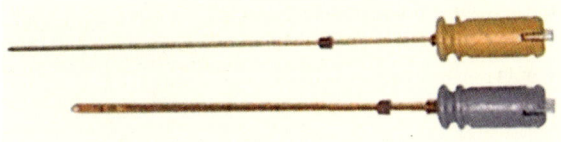

Fig. 8.11: Tips to instrument canals in posterior teeth

The Gordon group used a 200 micron diameter tip with radial emission; the maximum bactericidal power was reached at the maximum tested power (0.4 W, 20 Hz), with a 4-minute exposure time, without water in dry mode, with a bacterial eradication of 99.71%. The minimum time of irradiation of 15 sec with the minimum power (0.2 W, 20 Hz), with water spray, obtained 94.7% bacterial reduction.

The Schoop study examined parameters of 0.6 W and 0.9 W with a 200-micron fiber that produced a very contained thermal rise respectively of 1.3°C and 1.6°C, showing a high bactericidal effect on *E. coli* and *E. faecalis.*

Photo-activated Disinfection

Photo-activated disinfection is a unique combination of a photosensitizer solution and low-power laser light. The concept is internationally called **PACT (photodynamic antimicrobial chemotherapy), LAD (light-activated disinfection) or PAD (photo-activated disinfection).**

The *principle* on which it operates is that photosensitizer molecules attach to the membrane of the bacteria. Irradiation with light at a specific wavelength matched to the peak absorption of the photosensitizer leads to the production of singlet oxygen, which causes the bacterial cell wall to rupture killing the bacteria (Fig. 8.12).[86]

Using the principles described above, a system has been developed for endodontic use consisting of a small diode laser connected to a delivery fiber, disposable handpiece and

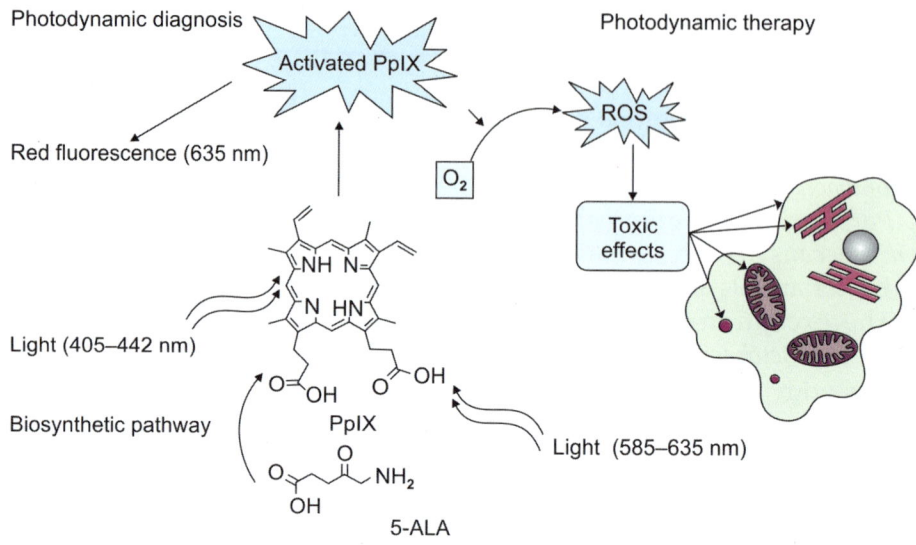

Fig. 8.12: Light of an appropriate energy (i.e. with a wavelength at the absorption maximum) is absorbed by protoporphyrin IX (PpIX), which undergoes a transition from a low-energy ground state to the excited singlet state. In photodynamic therapy, the activated photosensitizer interacts with oxygen to produce singlet oxygen and other radical species that cause a toxic effect in tumor cells or microorganisms. In photodynamic diagnosis, the illumination of PpIX (irradiated at a lower wavelength than in photodynamic therapy) leads to the emission of red fluorescence. ROS = reactive oxygen species; 5-ALA = 5-aminolevulinic acid

emitter. This is used in conjunction with a 12.7 mg/L solution of the photosensitiser, Tolonium chloride and indocyanine green.[86] It has been shown to be effective in killing the common bacteria associated with endodontic infections such as *Fusobacterium nucleatum*, *Prevotella intermedia*, *Streptococcus intermedius* and *Peptostreptococcus micros*. It has also been shown that the PAD system will kill *Enterococcus faecalis* which is regarded as one of the contaminants associated with canals which have recurrent infections (Fig. 8.13).

The emitter is a flexible hollow tube coated internally with a light diffusing material of a comparable size to the tip of an ISO standard #40 file. The light is emitted over a 15 mm length of the tip with a uniform energy density. This energy density is increased by 30% at the tip. After completion of canal preparation, the canal is inoculated with the

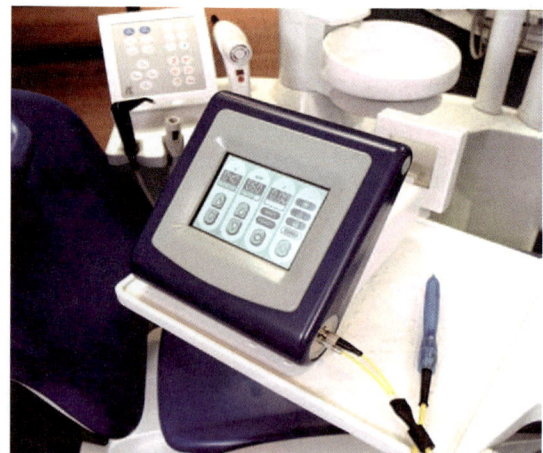

Fig. 8.13: The PAD unit—diode laser and endodontic handpiece

photosensitizer solution which is left in situ for a fixed period of time (60 seconds) to permit the solution to come into contact with the bacteria and diffuse through any biofilm

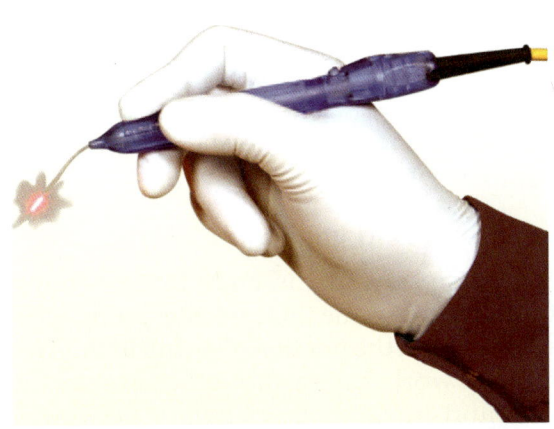

Fig. 8.14: Emitter handpiece and emitter

structure. The emitter is then placed in the root canal and irradiation carried out for 120 seconds. This has been demonstrated in the laboratory study to kill high concentrations of bacteria generally found in root canals (Fig. 8.14).[86]

Several factors affect the results created using PAD. These include the type of dye used, the dye concentration, the dose of radiation applied and the species of microorganism involved.

Dyes

Over 400 different photoactive dyes are known. Some of them are already used in dentistry:
- *Tolonium chloride (toluidine blue 0 or TBO)*
  - Aqueous solution
  - Sodium phosphate buffer
  - Peak absorption 633 nm
  - Dye concentration 12–100 mg/mL.
  - Radiation dose of typically 40 J/cm^2
  - Temperature of the dye is also an unknown factor and deserves further research
  - Long-term safety proven (oral carcinoma staining protocols with much higher doses, e.g. *Orascreen*)

- *Methylene blue*: Peak absorption 670 nm
- *Rose bengal*: Peak absorption 550 nm
- *Aluminum disulphonated phthalocyanine*: Peak absorption 675 nm
- *Parphyrin*
- *Polylysine*
- *Chlorine conjugated dyes*

PAD can be obtained with more than 400 photoactive substances, combined with different laser devices. Ten kinds of blue, purple and green dyes are the most effective and popular, mainly of the phenylmethane family. Blue seems to work the best and is best documented.

Radiation Dose

Several visible red semiconductor diode lasers are available:
- *SaveDent* diode laser (Denfotex Light Systems Ltd., Scotland), now commercially available as Aseptim™ PAD (SciCan, Germany): 635 nm, 50–100 mW with TBO + customized emitters.
- *Ceralase PDT* diode laser (CeramOptic, Germany): 662 nm, 0.5 W with chlorine dyes.
- *Biolitec* diode laser (Biolitec AG, Germany): 665 nm with chlorine dyes.
- *FOTO$_2$SAN* (CMS dental): 625–635 nm with TBO + customized emitters

Radiation doses are typically related to time, power, and energy density
- 40 J/cm^2
- Power 100 mW

Species of Microorganism

Virtually all microbial organisms can be inactivated by the right kind of PAD. In general, due to cell wall properties, Gram-positive pathogens are more sensitive to PAD than their Gram-negative counterparts. With PAD using TBO, this difference is marginal due to its cationic nature. *S. sobrinus, Lactobacillus casei, Actinomyces viscosus,* and *Veillonella* spp., main cariogenic micro-organisms can also be inactivated by PAD. Even in biofilms on carious dentine, kill rates of *S. mutans* were significant. Again, these rates were stronger in planktonic than in biofilm mode. There is a consistent lack of in vivo research. In the endodontic literature, *E. faecalis, S. intermedius, F. nucleatum, P. micros* and *P. intermedia* have been investigated regarding their sensitivity to PAD. All showed significant reductions in viable counts (Figs 8.15 and 8.16).

In 2005, Bonsor, Nichol, Reid and Pearson conducted an in vivo study to determine the microbiological effect of photo-activated disinfection (PAD) as an adjunct to normal root canal disinfection.[86] A microbiological sample of the canal was taken on accessing the canal, after conventional endodontic therapy and finally after PAD. All 3 samples from each canal were plated within 30 minutes of sampling and cultured anaerobically for 5 days and growth of viable bacteria was recorded for each sample to determine bacterial load. It was found that PAD system offers a means of destroying bacteria remaining after conventional irrigants in endodontic therapy.[86]

Laser-Activated Irrigation

Water, present in the endodontic irrigant solutions, limits the thermal interaction of the laser beam on the dentinal wall but at the same time can work synergistically when activated by a mid-infrared laser (water is a target chromophore) to clean the canal. In fact, irrigation is an essential part of root canal therapy because it allows for cleaning and bacterial reduction beyond what might be achieved by root canal instrumentation alone. Sodium hypochlorite (NaOCl) is the most commonly used root canal irrigant because it can dissolve organic tissue, kill micro-organisms, and act as a lubricant. However,

Actinomyces antinomycetemcomitans
Actinomyces naeslundii
Candida albicans
Enterococcus faecalis
Fusobacterium nucleatum
Pseudomonas aeruginosa
Prevotella intermedia
Prophyromonas gingivalis
Proteus mirabilis
Peptostreptococcus micros
Streptococcus intermedius
Sterptococcus mutans
Sterptococcus pyogenes
Sterptococcus sanguinis
Sterptococcus sobrinus

Fig. 8.15: Bacteria and fungi that respond to photo-dynamic antimicrobial chemotherapy (PACT)

Phenothiazine dyes	Methylene Bule
	Toluidine Blue O
Phthalocyanines	Aluminium disulfonated phthalocyanine
	Cationic Zn(II)-phthalocyanine
Chlorines	Chlorin e6
	Sn(IV) chlorin e6
	Chlorin e6-2.5 N-methyl-D-glucamine
	Polylysine and polyethyleneimine conjugates of chlorin e6
Porphyrins	Hematoporphyrin HCl
	Aminolevulinic acid
	Photofrin (dihematoporphyrin ether)
Xanthenes	Erythrosine
Monoterpenes	Azulene

Fig. 8.16: Photosensitizers applied in PACT

because of high surface tension, sodium hypochlorite penetrates only 130 μm into dentinal tubules, while bacteria can colonize the dentinal tubules deeply up to the periodontal surface (1100 μm from the canal lumen). Lasers have been recently proposed to activate irrigation solutions by the transfer of pulsed energy.

Laser activation of solutions occurs primarily by photomechanical and photothermal mechanisms, rather than by photochemical or photodynamic processes. For endodontic irrigants, the alkaline- or acid-etching effects of irrigants are enhanced by agitation of the fluids in the canal. This agitation allows better penetration of fluids into the nooks and crannies of the complex root canal anatomy. An increase in temperature will also occur, which will accelerate chemical reactions, such as etching and dissolution of proteins.

By causing intense agitation, the erbium *laser-generated shockwaves (LGS)* enhance the action of root canal irrigants, including ethylene diamine tetra-acetic acid (EDTA), to provide effective removal of dense smear layers.

High temperature and agitation were shown to enhance the efficacy of sodium hypochlorite; the effect of agitation on tissue dissolution was reportedly greater than that of temperature, with continuous agitation of sodium hypochlorite resulting in the fastest tissue dissolution.

With near- and mid-infrared lasers, some level of temperature increase in the fluid will occur, and this will contribute to the overall effect, above and beyond the effect caused by LGS. The ability of LGS to debride the canal depends upon the efficiency of the energy absorption within the fluid; the energy, shape, and duration of the laser pulse; and the power density achieved at the fiber tip. Changing the shape of the fiber tip influences the direction of the shockwaves so that they can be

predominantly targeted on to the walls of the root canal. In contrast, the LGS produced by a plain fiber primarily travels in a forward direction, and thus is largely parallel to the walls of the root canal surface to be ablated, resulting in lower efficiency.

The following technical issues influence the selection of systems for LGS-based methods in endodontics:

1. For effective LGS using aqueous fluids, the laser wavelength chosen must be absorbed in water. LGS have been shown with erbium (Er:YAG and Er, Cr:YSGG), 940 and 980 nm diode, and Nd:YAG lasers. For the diode lasers, the LGS effect can be enhanced by including a low concentration of hydrogen peroxide in the fluid. This changes the absorption profile, and also generates a secondary cavitation bubble from the production of oxygen.

2. A conventional plain fiber tip will deliver laser energy primarily in a forward direction (parallel to the fiber tip), with limited lateral emissions.

3. The flexibility of fiberoptic delivery systems (regardless of the material used) reduces as their diameter increases. Furthermore, fibers require a larger arc to attain a degree of flexibility comparable to that of nickel titanium (NiTi) instruments, thus making fibers stiffer and more difficult to use in highly curved canals.

4. High transmission losses are seen with fiberoptics used with erbium lasers. Passage of laser energy through fiberoptics can undergo attenuation, which may be dependent on the absorption characteristics of the fiber. In the mid-infrared range, quartz glass fibers have a much lower transmissibility than sapphire. Tran reported that quartz fibers transmit very poorly at wavelengths above 2.5 microns, thus for an Er:YAG laser only 30% of the

laser power can be transmitted through a quartz tip which is 12 mm long. For wavelengths in the mid-infrared regions, conventional quartz glass fibers may be used provided a doping agent, such as fluoride or germanium is included to increase the transmission efficiency of the fiber.

5. Fiber diameter influences the requirement for minimal preparation before the fiber can be inserted to the required point. At the present time, 200 micron fibers are commonly used, hence canals need to be widened to the minimum size of an ISO #20 file before the fiber can be used safely in the root canal.

6. Fibers with a plain end have right angles at their tips which tend to bind on to the canal walls, and restrict the smooth movement of the fiber toward the apex in curved canals.

7. Unlike stainless steel hand endodontic files, optical fiber tips cannot be precurved to the canal shape. The tendency of the fiber to return to its lowest energy position (i.e. being straight) forces it to push against the canal wall, giving an inherent risk of ledges or perforations during withdrawal of a flexible fiber. Such fibers will straighten past the curve, and the emitted energy will be delivered directly on to the location on the wall of the canal that has the least curvature.

8. Conventional plain optical fibers, unlike hand or rotary endodontic instruments, have parallel sides, which makes them prone to frictional binding in the canal, particularly in the apical third of the canal.

The ablative effect of lasers on hard tissues, such as dentin, is influenced by a number of factors, including:

• Water film thickness
• Pulse energy
• Beam diameter
• Pulse duration

Erbium laser systems have pulse durations which can be classified as:

a. Long pulse (e.g. above 500 microseconds)
b. Short pulse (typically 200–400 microseconds), and
c. Very short pulse (less than 200 microseconds).

In addition, the LGS effect and the pattern of ablation are both influenced by the shape of the fiber tip. Fiber tips with sculpted polished ends and greater lateral emissions have been developed in an attempt to overcome some of the problems related to plain fiber designs.

FIBEROPTICS AND THEIR MODIFICATIONS

For a laser to be useful in endodontics, it must be able to effectively deliver laser energy to the root canal of both anterior and posterior teeth. Fiberoptics were introduced into medicine in 1954 by Hopkins and Kapany.

Optical fibers work by total internal reflection, and in general comprise three concentric layers. Light passes only through the central glass core of the fiber. This is surrounded by a cladding, which has a lower refractive index than the core. The cladding layer may be doped with different materials, such as fluoride, to alter its refractive index. The outer layer is the buffer layer and is used only for mechanical strength and protection of the fiber. The buffer coating is normally a polymer material, such as polyvinylchloride.

The most commonly used material to fabricate fibers is quartz glass or fused silica,

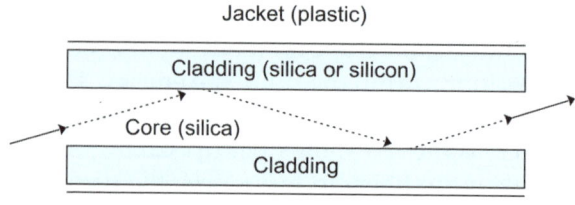

Fig. 8.17

either in a pure form or with one or more dopants added, such as fluoride, phosphate, and germanium. These dopants added to the core act as transmitters or amplifiers, which overcome to some extent the expected losses. Recently, fibers doped with rare earth elements or other dopants have emerged as a promising medium. Fibers can also be fabricated from a range of non-glass crystalline materials, including rare earth oxides and minerals such as sapphire, as well as from ceramics or polymers.

Although quartz tips have high transmission losses in the infrared range, their better physical properties make them the popular choice for delivering laser energy within the root canal.

The advantages of optical fibers over other delivery systems are their small size and high flexibility. Sapphire fibers transmit some light wavelengths better than quartz, sapphire fibers are rigid, often rupture on bending, and can only be polished not cleaved, making shaping the tips much more difficult. Moreover, unlike quartz fibers, crystalline sapphire cannot be reheated to produce different shapes by drawing out the fiber. Sapphire fibers are more expensive than glass fibers because the growth process is much slower than the glass fiber drawing process.

De Moor et al also examined the effects of laser activation of irrigants, comparing it to conventional irrigation (CI) and to passive ultrasound irrigation (PUI). In their study, an Er,Cr:YSGG laser was used, 4 times for 5 seconds at 75 mJ, 20 Hz (1.5 W) with an endodontic tip (200-micron diameter, with flat tip), held steady at 5 mm from the apex, to activate sodium hypochlorite at 2.5%. The removal of the smear layer performed with this procedure resulted in significantly better results with respect to the other two methods. It was not necessary to move the fiber up and down in the canal, but was sufficient to keep it steady in the middle third at 5 mm from the apex. This concept greatly simplifies the laser technique, without the need to approach the apex and to negotiate radicular curves.

METHODS OF MODIFYING TIPS

Fiber tips are commonly modified by pulling or by chemical etching. Alternatively, the fiber end can be polished. A flat surface can be polished at an angle to accommodate a totally reflecting surface for a unidirectional side-firing fiber. If the fiber tip is rotated while being polished at a small angle, a tapered tip will result, with multidirectional emissions.

The tip can also be modified by fixing certain materials to the fiber end to disperse the light across wide angles. Such tips are commonly called *isotropic tips* and are widely used in photodynamic therapy. However, these tips can only be used at relatively low energy levels.

Chemical Etching

A typical chemical etching process involves immersing a fiberoptic tip into a solution of etchant covered with an insoluble organic solvent. The chemical composition most commonly used for etching is 40–50% hydrofluoric acid (HF), topped with silicone oil. The oil not only prevents emissions of harmful HF vapors, but also modifies the contact angle between the fiber and the etchant.

Inorganic solvents including isooctane, 1-bromodecane, and 1-octanethiol may be used as alternatives to silicone oil. Etching is typically done in polystyrene containers which are chemically resistant to HF.

It is the simplest and most inexpensive method of shaping the tip to obtain a conical end which gives a broad distribution of energy, while still allowing for high optical transmission.

There are several different methods within which etching is used to modify fibers, including:

- Static and dynamic etching, and
- Tube etching which is used for polymer-coated materials.

Modified Tip Profiles

Two important factors that influence the characteristics of the laser energy passing through any fiber are the refractive index of the fiber material and the diameter of the fiber. The geometry and optical properties of fibers define their possible applications.

Clarkin et al[61] and Verdaasdonk et al[62] have described various shaped tips (e.g. ball-ended, tapered, shielded, metal-coated). Shoji et al[42] described a conical tip with a fan-shaped emission profile, delivering 80 percent of the energy laterally, and only 20 percent in the forward direction, while Heisterkamp et al[63] used cylindrical diffusion tips for coagulating solid tumors, however, their size (diameter 1.65 mm) is too large for endodontic applications.

Ideally, lasers to be used in endodontics for smear layer removal, canal shaping, and disinfection should employ fiberoptic tips which are *side-firing* so that they can deliver laser energy laterally on to the canal walls. The tip design should also prevent unwanted effects of the laser past the apical foramen.

Spherical and cylindrical tips with a near-360-degree emission profile *(isotropic tips)* have been used for photo-activated disinfection of root canals using low-intensity visible red light, but the designs are not suited to delivering high-intensity pulses in the near-(780–1400 nm) and mid-infrared (1400–3000 nm) ranges.

An alternative method of achieving a 360-degree emission profile is using embedded

titanium dioxide which can disperse near-infrared laser energy laterally along the length of the fiber tip; however, such tips are expensive and are too large (0.6 mm) for clinical use in endodontics.

Other variants of tips are conical and patterned conical (honeycomb) tips as well as safe-tipped variants of same technology.

These "safe" tips used silver plating to reduce emission of laser energy in the forward direction.

Such fiber tip surface modifications increase emissions on to the walls of the root canal, and allow for greater control of the LGS effect created by cavitation events which occur along the surface of the tip. For example, conical honeycomb tips with safe ends can activate fluids placed in the root canal and generate shockwaves that are directed on to the walls of the root canals and also into lateral canals, deltas, and isthmus areas.

A further advantage of these tip designs is that they are simpler to use in practice because it is no longer necessary for the operator to follow complex sequences of moving and withdrawing the fiber in order to achieve even irradiation of the canal walls, as is currently undertaken with conventional or radial firing tips.

In terms of their therapeutic applications, modified tips which have a conical shape offer particular advantages in endodontics. The tip shape alters the LGS effect and helps guide the fiber into narrow regions of the canal. In 2008, George et al reported that a conical tip could enhance the removal of the smear layer in the root canal over a conventional plain tip. The improved LGS effect obtained with either Er:YAG or Er,Cr:YSGG lasers improves the action of EDTA with Cetavlon (EDTAC) and other aqueous irrigants.

Recently, a variation on the LGS concept known as *photon-induced photoacoustic streaming* (PIPS) has been introduced, which uses more rigid, short conical tips as opposed to flexible tips with long conical ends. It presupposes the use of an Er:YAG laser (LightWalker AT, Fotona, Ljubljana, Slovenia) and its interaction with irrigant solutions (sodium hypochlorite, EDTA, distilled water)[18–20,36] differently from the preceding LAI.

PIPS® was developed by Dr. Enrico DiVito, along with his research team at Medical Dental Advanced Technologies Group, LLC (MDATG) with assistance from Dr. Mark Colonna.

A novel nonablative, 9 mm long, 600 µm diameter quartz tapered tip with the polyamide sheath stripped 3 mm from its end is used with an erbium: yttrium-aluminum-garnet (Er:YAG) laser to deliver shock waves throughout the root canal system. Photon-induced photoacoustic streaming (PIPS) uses extremely low energy levels (< 20 mJ) and short microsecond pulse rates (50 µs at a wavelength of 2,940 nm) to create peak power spikes that generate a profound shock wave which travels three-dimensionally throughout the root canal system (Fig. 8.18).

This technique uses more of the photo-acoustic and photomechanical phenomena rather than the photothermal.

The use of low-energy (20 mJ at 15 Hz, 0.3 W average power, or less) generates a minimal thermal effect. Erbium laser energy is delivered at only 50 microsecond pulse duration through a specially designed, tapered and stripped, 600 micron diameter, 9 mm long tip (LightWalker, Fotona, Ljubljana-Slovenia), it produces a high peak power of 400 Watts when compared to a longer pulse duration. Each impulse, absorbed by the water molecules, creates a strong "shock wave" that leads to the formation of an effective streaming of fluids inside the canal while also avoiding side effects seen with other methodologies.

The profound and distant effect of PIPS™ eliminates the need to introduce the tip into the root canal system. Unlike traditional laser techniques requiring placement of the tip 1 mm from the apex, or even 5 mm from the apex as proposed for LAI, the PIPS™ tip is placed only in the coronal portion of the pulpal chamber and left stationary, allowing the photoacoustic waves to spread into the openings of each canal (Figs 8.19 and 8.20).

A new tip design consisting of a 600 micron diameter, 9 millimeter long tapered end is used for this technique. The final 3 millimeters of coating is stripped from the end to allow for greater lateral emission of energy

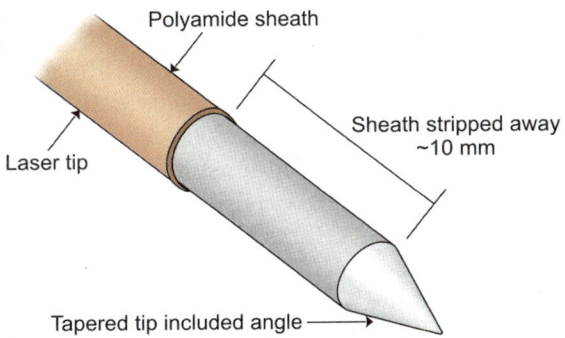

Fig. 8.18: This image depicts the novel 9 mm long, 600 µm diameter quartz tapered photon-induced photoacoustic streaming (PIPS) tip with the polyamide sheath stripped 3 mm from its end

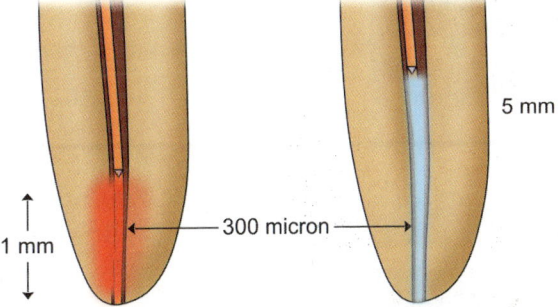

Fig. 8.19: Position of the laser fibers in the traditional laser endodontic technique: 1 mm short of the apex (left) and in LAI (right), 5 mm short of the apex

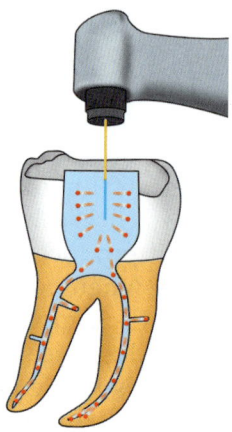 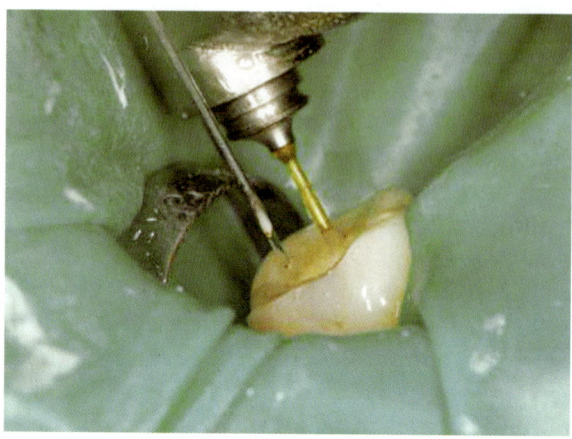

Fig. 8.20: PIPS™ technique: The tip must be placed in the coronal chamber with open access to the canals

compared to the frontal tip. This mode of energy emission allows for improved lateral diffusion of the low energy, enhanced photoacoustic waves (Fig. 8.21).

This mode of energy emission makes better use of the laser energy when, at subablative levels, it is delivered with very high nominal peak powers for each single pulse of 50 microseconds (400 W). This in turn produces powerful shock waves in the irrigants leading to a demonstrable and significant mechanical effect on the dentinal wall.

Results from as-yet-unpublished fluid dynamics studies from the University of

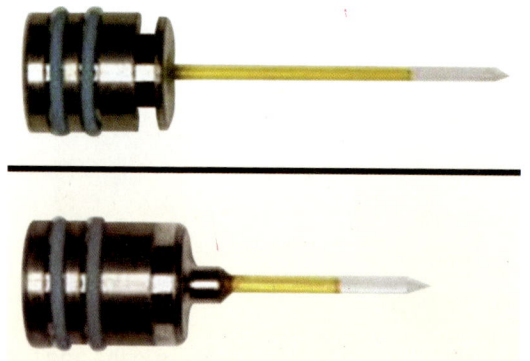

Fig. 8.21: PIPS 400/12 and 600/9 tips

Southern California demonstrate significant differences in velocities and movement when ultrasonic irrigation was compared to PIPS. Ultrasonic analysis showed a more "linear" and standing wave-type of fluid movement which was located only within 0.5 to 1.0 mm of the tip. Activity was measured at distances in 3 mm increments from the tip to 21 mm and no significant movement was seen past 3 mm. PIPS on the other hand showed a more dramatic "turbulent" flow movement when compared to the use of ultrasonic. Of particular interest was the ability of this technique to show significant movement not only near the tip, but distant from the tip. At 21 mm, the velocities achieved with PIPS were 4 times greater than those with the ultrasonic device. This makes PIPS a useful irrigation tool for the clinician to more effectively move and drive irrigants three-dimensionally to all the smaller and complex dental morphologies often seen in the difficult-to-reach apical third and also allows for cleaning and bacterial reduction of the root canal efficiently without the need to enlarge the apical preparation. This ultimately leads to improving the success rate of therapies in both narrow and curved canals without the need to enlarge the apical preparation, contributing to a more minimally invasive preparation and methodology.

Few studies have investigated the ability of lasers to remove bacterial biofilm from canal walls. Bacterial biofilm is a thin layer of microorganisms in which cells adhere to each other on a surface, frequently embedded within a self-generated matrix of extracellular polymeric substance that protect them from chemical and physical forces. In contrast, planktonic cells of the same organism are single cells that may float or swim in a liquid medium and may be easily destroyed by chemical irrigants or lasers. Peters et al reported a significant reduction of the bacterial load of 99.5% of 3 week-incubated bacterial biofilm, by using PIPS and NaOCl for 30 seconds with 30 seconds of resting time. Pedulla et al also reported a strong reduction of bacterial load of 99.8% of *Enterococcus faecalis* cells incubated for 15 days by using

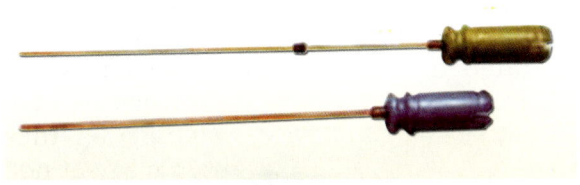

Fig. 8.22: Z2 and Z3 endo tips (200 and 300 microns) for an Er,Cr:YSGG laser

30 seconds of Er:YAG laser activation. This study also indicated that laser activation of distilled water alone was not sufficient to yield bacteria reduction (73%); this report underscored the role of sodium hypochlorite in root canal disinfection but also the importance of physical impact of the shock wave in bacterial cell destruction.

In recent years, a new protocol has been developed that addresses also the second disadvantage of classically performed root-canal treatments that is complete mechanical preparation of the complex side canal system, as well as the complete removal of the smear layer. For the effective debridement and cleaning of the complex root-canal system, the extremely high absorption of the pulsed Er:YAG laser wavelength at 2,940 nm in water and chemical rinsing is utilized to create a "cleansing" photoacoustic effect within the root-canal system as a laser-assisted irrigation (LAI). The Er:YAG laser pulses are emitted from a thin side-firing endo tip, so they are immediately fully absorbed by the rinsing, creating shock waves that mechanically debride the root-canal system with a minimal thermal impact on the dentin. It results in a complete removal of the smear layer with open dentinal tubules and an intact collagen structure, performing also a biomodulation of the fibroblasts and preparing the root-canal

Table 8.3: Intracanal laser techniques					
Laser technique	*Laser effect*	*Tip position*	*Tip size*	*Tip design*	*Apical preparation*
Direct radiation	Photothermal	Apex 1 mm shorter	200–300 microns	End firing	ISO 30–40
LAI	Photothermal, cavitation	Middle third 5 mm shorter	200–400 microns	Tapered or chemically modified	ISO 30–40
PIPS	Photothermal, Photoacoustic, photomechanical, shock wave	Pulp chamber	400 micron	Tapered or stripped	ISO 20–25

Table 8.4: Summary of laser techniques in endodontics

Laser technique	Laser energy (mJ)	Pulse duration (microseconds)	Nominal peak power (watts)	Fiber (microns)	Fiber position	Apical preparation	Erbium laser wave-length (nm)
LAI 10 × 5 sec	37.5	140, 200	267 187	400 Conically modified	WL less 1mm	ISO 50/5 Working length	2780, 2940
LAI 4 × 5 sec	75	140 250	535 300	200	WL less 5 mm	ISO 40/6 Working length	2780 2940
LAI 1 min	65	250	260	280	WL less 1 mm, moved up and down × 4 mm	0.23 mm	2940
LAI	11 18 26	250	44 72 104	300 Cone shaped	WL less 2 mm or 5 mm stationary	1 mm	2940
PIPS 20–40 sec	20	50	400	400 PIPS	Pulp chamber, stationary	ISO 20/.06	2940

network for an almost perfect 3D filling (Fig.8.23).

Known as the Twinlight™ Endodontic Treatment (TET) as proposed by Dr. Norbert Guktnecht of University of Aachen is based on Fotona Twinlight complimentary laser wavelengths concept. This new protocol involves two complementary "gold" standard wavelengths: the deeply penetrating Nd:YAG laser wavelength for the deep thermal disinfection of the dentin, and the highly absorbed Er:YAG laser wavelength for the non-thermal, photoacoustic cleaning and debridement of the complex root canal system, accompanied by an efficient biomodulation of fibroblasts (Fig. 8.24).

The TET procedure consists of three laser treatment steps: First, the sophisticated hard-tissue ablative capability of the Er:YAG laser allows a selective and pressure-free, less painful access to the pulp chamber, decontaminating the area and ablating the irritated tissue. The bacterial load is not

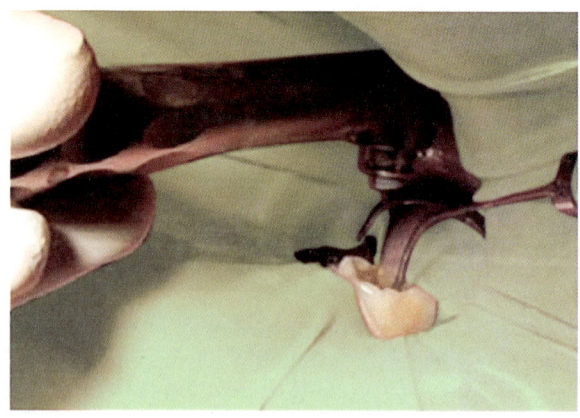

Fig. 8.23: Removal of debris and smear layer from root canals using the Er:YAG laser. The treatment is accompanied by collateral irrigation with saline solution

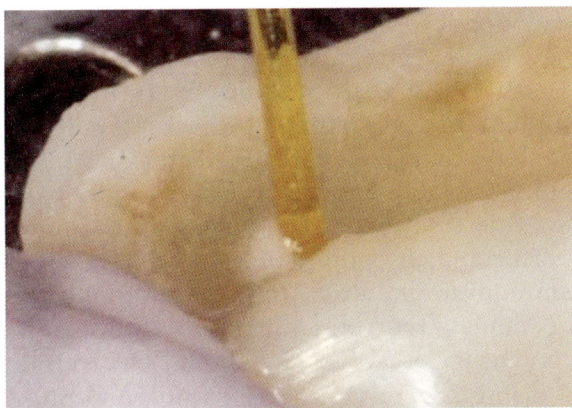

Fig. 8.24: *Deep decontamination with Nd:YAG laser (3–5 times per session)*

pushed into deeper root areas, significantly reducing the danger of spreading of the bacterial wave throughout the body system.

Secondly, the root-canal system is cleaned and debrided with Er:YAG-induced photo-acoustics. Two protocols are being used for this procedure, either Preciso side-firing tips with saline solution at 20–65 mJ and 15–25 Hz, or alternatively PIPS radial-firing tips at 10–20 mJ and 10–50 Hz with EDTA (15–17%) as rinsing.

During the third step, the root canal is rinsed, dried, and deeply decontaminated using the Nd:YAG 200 ìm laser fiber at 1.5 W and 15 Hz.

Twinlight™ procedure represents an endodontic therapy that successfully addresses both factors that complicate achieving sterility in the tooth: the anatomical root configuration and characteristics of deeply resident bacterial flora.

Twinlight™ approach represents a progressive decontamination from the first to the last step of laser assisted endodontics. It reduces the risk of bacteria spreading into perioperative area of the body system which is particularly important for immune

compromised patients. It also produces three dimensional root canal wall anatomy with open and decontaminated dentin tubules.

In conclusion, the combination of two laser wavelengths comes very close to being a truly "universal" dental laser system.

Lasers are making significant contributions to every step in the practice of endodontics, from diagnosis using Doppler flowmeter technology to preventive measures involving pulp capping and pulpotomy. Lasers may be used for cleaning, disinfecting, and obturating root-canal systems. When conventional endodontic therapy fails, **laser-assisted endodontic retreatment** is now a viable treatment alternative.

The objective of non-surgical retreatment is to eliminate from the root canal space sources of irritation to the attachment apparatus.[44] The rationale for using laser irradiation in non-surgical retreatment may be ascribed to the need to remove foreign material from the root-canal system that may be otherwise difficult to remove by conventional methods.[44]

The **neodymium: yttrium-aluminum-perovskite (Nd:YAP) laser** emitting at 1340 nm (Blum and Abadie, 1997, Farge et al, 1998) was suggested as an effective device for root-canal preparation in endodontic retreatment (200 mJ and a frequency of 10 Hz).[44]

Yu et al used an Nd:YAG laser at three output powers (1, 2 and 3 W) to remove gutta-percha and broken files from root canals. They were able to remove filling material in more than 70% of samples while broken files were removed in 55% samples.[44]

The efficacy of Er:YAG laser in removing zinc-oxide sealers and phenoplastic resins has also been studied. In straight root canals, laser irradiation with 250 mJ/pulse and 10 Hz frequency was useful in eliminating zinc-oxide sealers.[44]

A clinical advantage that should be further explored is the possibility of eliminating the use of toxic solvents when removing semi-solid materials from root canals. Although, it has been shown that root canal filling material can be removed using lasers, such as Nd:YAG and Er:YAG, the decisive advantage in using lasers for this purpose still remains to be confirmed.[44]

During endodontic treatment, accidental perforation of pulp-chamber wall by a cutting instrument may occur. Based on anatomic location, **pulp chamber perforations** can be divided into gingival and periodontal membrane types. The periodontal membrane type is further divided into pulp chamber floor, apical and lateral root canal wall sub-types of these, perforations of pulp-chamber floor is extremely difficult to treat and studies have shown that the prognosis is markedly worse when compared to other types of perforations.[134]

The basic treatment is to sterilize the affected area (removal of smear layer) and form an air-tight seal.[134]

It was shown that Nd:YAG laser was effective in removing the smear layer and this aided in healing of apical lesions because the smear layer containing organic components was reduced in volume. Also, it has a small coefficient for tissue absorption, penetrates deep into the tissue and is capable of heat coagulation of capillary networks in tissue; as a result, it shows excellent hemostasis.[134]

Thus it was concluded that pulp-chamber floor perforations can be effectively treated by eliminating the smear-layer using Nd:YAG laser and polymerizing the light-cured composite resin using argon laser.[134]

Pulpless teeth have a tendency to fracture. Many dentists encounter at least one case in which they are obliged to extract a tooth because of fracture despite finishing the

endodontic treatment.[42] To prevent such cases, new laser techniques are being developed. Teeth lased with 38% silver ammonium solution became difficult to fracture. Pulpless teeth are indicated for this treatment. Pulsed Nd:YAG, CO_2, and argon lasers can be used for this treatment. The laser irradiation is performed in combination with 38% silver ammonium solution until the tooth surface becomes silver and mirror-like under air-cooling at 2 or 3 W and for about 20 seconds.[42]

Using a neodymium: yttrium-aluminum-garnet laser beam to **seal vertical root fracture** line with tricalcium phosphate paste represents an alternative treatment for cracked teeth with noted clinical results. Levy and Koubi, G.F.(1993) studied the permeability of molten crystals of hydroxyapatite in the dentin of a cracked root after crack lines have been filled with a preparation of tricalcium phosphate melted by a neodymium: yttrium-aluminum-garnet laser beam. The morphology of the sealed cracks was analyzed under a scanning electron microscope that showed a deep fusion of tricalcium phosphate along crack lines.[82]

Lin C.P., Lin F.H., et al (2000) tried to use a developed DP-bioactive glass paste to fuse or bridge the tooth crack line by a medium energy continuous-wave CO_2 laser. Their study was divided into three parts:
1. The compositional and structure changes in tooth enamel and dentin after laser treatment;
2. The phase transformation and re-crystallization of DP-bioactive paste during exposure to the CO_2 laser; and
3. The thermal interactions and bridge mechanism between DP-bioactive glass paste and enamel/dentin when they are subjected to CO_2 laser. They examined the changes of laser-exposed DP-bioactive glass paste by means of X-ray diffractometer

(XRD), Fourier transforming infrared spectroscopy (FTIR), differential thermal analysis/thermogravimetric analysis (DTA/TGA), and scanning electron microscopy (SEM).[82]

From the study, they found that the temperature increase due to laser irradiation was greater than 900°C and that the DP-bioactive glass paste could be melted in a short period of time after irradiation. In the study, they successfully developed a DP-bioactive glass paste, which could form a melting glass within seconds after exposure to a medium energy density continuous-wave CO_2 laser. The paste will be used in the near future to bridge the enamel or dentin surface crack by the continuous-wave CO_2 laser.[42]

As a last resort to prevent extraction of a tooth, lasers may be used in **apical surgery** to seal the root end of the tooth to prevent bacteria from entering the root-canal system. As this technology matures, more uses and perhaps more wavelengths will deliver superior endodontic care.

The first attempt to use a laser in endodontic surgery was performed by *Dr. Weichman* at the University of Southern California. He attempted to seal the apical foramen of extracted teeth from which pulps had been extirpated.[40]

The apices of these specimens were irradiated using a high-power CO_2 laser. Melting of cementum and dentin was observed with a "cap" formation.[40]

Miserendino used a CO_2 laser to irradiate the apex of tooth during apicectomy. The advantages associated with laser application for periapical surgery are improved hemostasis and concurrent visualization of operative field. The potential sterilizing effect of contaminated root apex as well as reduction in permeability of dentin was also emphasized.

Duclos et al used a CO_2 laser to perform apicoectomies in patients and advocated the use of a mini contra-angle head for efficient delivery of laser irradiation at a 90° angle to the root apices of posterior teeth. [46] Recently, it has been reported that when using an Er:YAG laser in a low-output power in apical surgery, it was possible to resect the apex of extracted teeth. Smooth and clean resected surfaces devoid of charring were observed. [133]

Advantages

- Absence of discomfort and vibration.
- Less chances of contamination at the surgical site.
- Reduced risk of trauma to adjacent tissues.

Gouw-Soares et al reported a new protocol for use in apical surgery:

Er:YAG	: Osteotomy and root resection
Nd:YAG	: To seal the dentinal tubules
GaAlAs diode laser	: To improve healing

Radiographic follow-up showed significant decrease in radioluscency around periapical areas with no adverse signs and symptoms.[133]

Appropriate wavelength to melt hard tissues of tooth has been established which is the main contribution of laser technology to surgical endodontics. It helps converting the apical dentin and cementum structure into a uniformity glazed area that does not allow egress of microorganisms through dentinal tubules and other openings in the apex of tooth. Hemostasis and sterilization of contaminated root apex will have additional input.[28]

Other future uses of lasers in endodontics foreseen are

- Removal of calcified attached denticle by pulsed dye laser (λ = 504 nm) {Rocca et al, 1994}.[141]

- To sterilize endodontic instruments using argon, CO_2 and Nd:YAG lasers.[141]

- Laser treatment of periapical lesions of sinus tract.[141]

With the development of thinner, more flexible and durable laser fibers, laser applications in endodontics will increase. Since laser devices are still relatively costly, access to them is limited. Ideally, the laser in the future will have the ability to produce a multitude of wavelengths and pulse widths, each specific to a particular application. Once our knowledge of optimal laser parameters for each treatment modality is complete, lasers can be developed that will provide dentists with the ability to care for patients with improved techniques.

9

Esthetics and Lasers

In this ever-changing world of fast-paced communication, marketing, and shared intelligence, the appearance or looks of someone or something can "make or break" the end result. Whether we peruse on-line, at the bookstore, at our favorite clothing store, or at a new job interview, the way that we look can have a major impact on acceptance and its end result.[144] It has been well documented that looking good can enhance social, romantic, and economic consequences and allow an attractive person to get a better job. It now is universally accepted that looking good directly affects an individual's self-confidence and the image that he or she conveys. Because the face and mouth are the most noticeable parts of the human body, it is no wonder that there is such an increase in demand for smile and teeth makeovers in everyday dental practices.[144] *"Esthetic" or "cosmetic" dentistry* is none other than restorative general dentistry completed to a level that simply makes every attempt to mimic a natural look. Moving from the "mechanical age" to the "adhesive age" in dentistry has forced practitioners to view teeth in an entirely different context. The profession also is seeing a change in the way gingival tissue is handled: with regard to gingival sculpting, it is seeing a move from the *"steel (scalpel) age"* to the *"laser age."* It now is possible, thanks to lasers, to alter gingival tissue conservatively to create a more natural, symmetric, and harmonious appearance.[144]

1. GINGIVECTOMY FOR TISSUE HYPERPLASIA

The laser (CO_2, diode) is used to incise the location of desired gingival margin in a

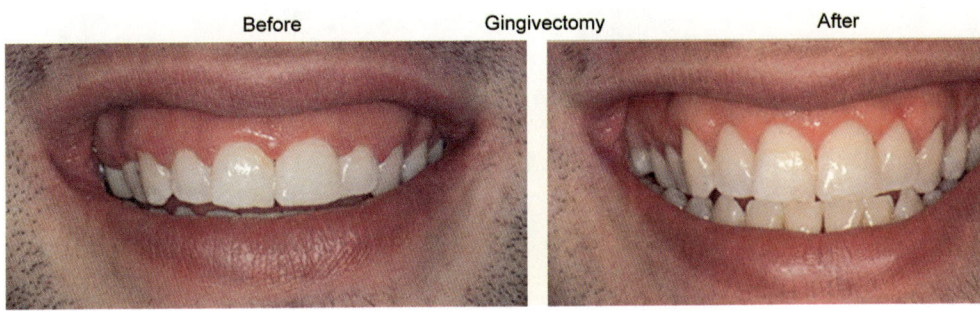

Before   Gingivectomy   After

Fig. 9.1

focused mode and then either to excise or ablate the superfluous hyperplastic tissues.[128]

Advantages

- Lack of bleeding.
- More precise control than electro-surgery.
- Lack of need of postoperative periodontal dressing.

2. GINGIVAL COSMETIC RESCULPTURING

In cases involving asymmetry of gingival tissues or excessive gingival tissue in isolated area, the laser (CO_2 or diode) can be used precisely sculpt the tissues to ideal contour. This is also a useful technique when papillary hypertrophy has occurred after orthodontic therapy or when an unesthetic papilla requires recontouring (Figs 9.2 to 9.4).[128]

The laser is used in focused mode and is aimed vertically down the tooth surface towards the tissue to avoid contact with the tooth surface.[128]

A slow to medium pulsed mode (2 to 10 pulses/second) enhances precision and allows the dentist to slowly run along the gingival margin and vertically remove the amount of tissue needed to obtain a desirable contour.[128]

3. FRENECTOMY (Fig. 9.5)

Most commonly used lasers are CO_2, diode, argon and Nd:YAG. The frenum can be

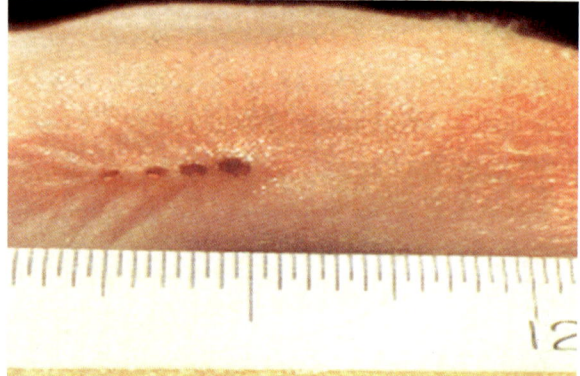

Fig. 9.2: Example of relative wound contracture occurring from various CO_2 laser exposures in the skin of a nude mouse

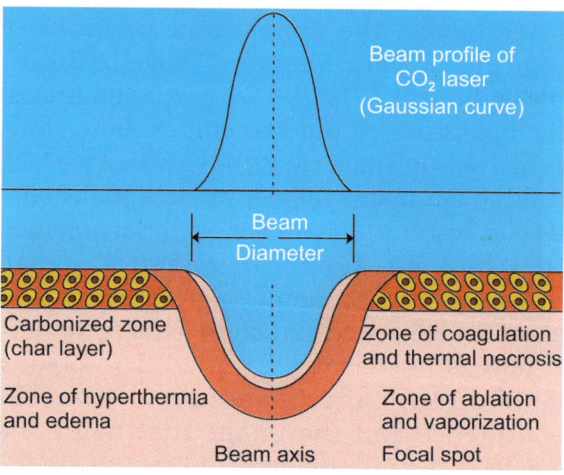

Fig. 9.3: Laser crater, shown is the relationship between beam profile and the crater produced in tissue by the CO_2 laser

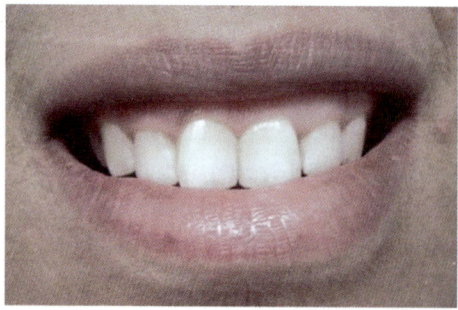
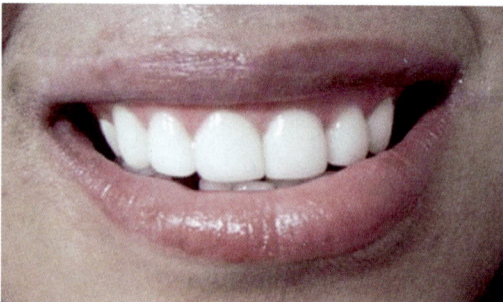

Fig. 9.4: Before and after gingival cosmetic resculpturing

excised in continuous, focused mode (or with a contact tip) or ablated in continuous or pulsed, defocused mode.[113]

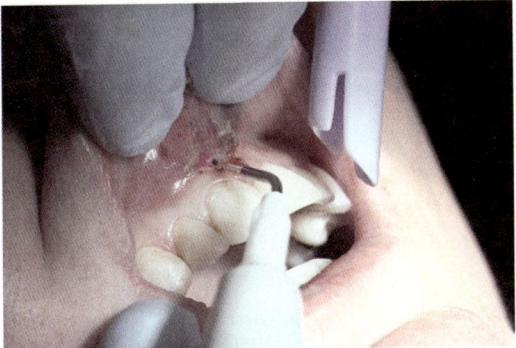

Before lingual frenectomy

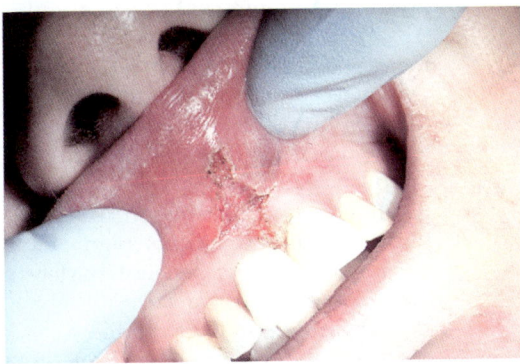

After lingual frenectomy

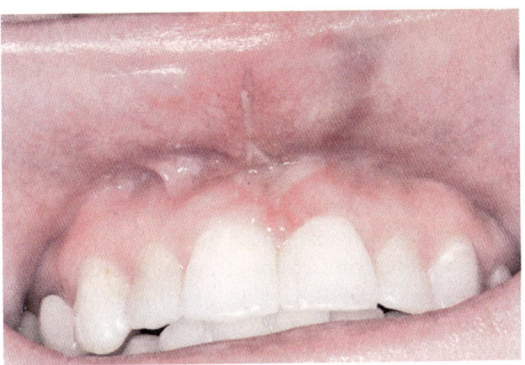

After 2 years

Fig. 9.5: Lingual frenectomy

Advantages

- Healing is excellent and no closure is necessary.
- Lack of bleeding and elimination of suture– an ideal technique for children.
- Sometimes can be performed without local unesthetic unless frenum is small.

4. GINGIVAL TROUGHING (Fig. 9.6)

The CO_2 and diode lasers are useful in bloodless gingival troughing before taking impressions. This eliminates the need for retraction cords and vasoconstrictors.[113]

The laser tip is placed below the height of gingival crevice and the tissue is "ledged" to expose the margin of preparation.[113]

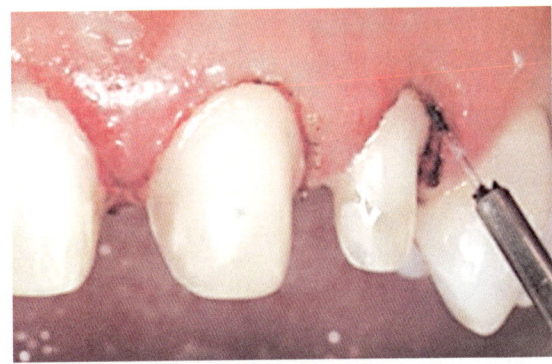

Laser positioning for gingival troughing

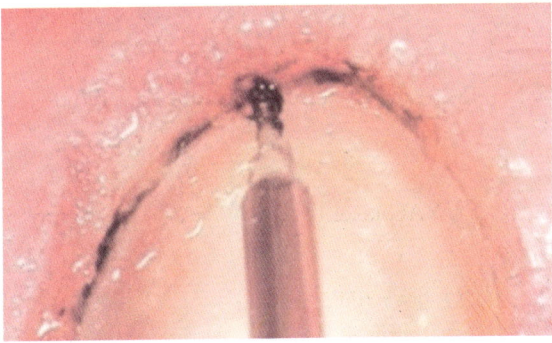

Close up of laser positioning

Fig. 9.6: Gingival troughing

Laser positioning for gingival troughing. Close up of laser positioning.

The procedure is technique-sensitive and must be done carefully to prevent in advertent damage to the tooth.[128]

5. LASER BLEACHING

The desire to have whiter teeth and the bleaching techniques have been documented since the mid-19th century. Laser-assisted bleaching has been introduced in an attempt to accelerate the bleaching process. Laser bleaching officially started in 1966 with approval of Ion Laser Technology's argon and carbon dioxide lasers by FDA.[53]

Types of Lasers Commonly used (Table 9.1)

Argon, carbon dioxide, Nd:YAG and Er, Cr: YSGG lasers are commonly used. Other lasers

Table 9.1: Types of lasers commonly used

Sr. no	Laser	Wavelength	Properties and risks
1.	Argon (CW or pulsed)	488 nm (blue)	Limited penetration depth into dental hard tissue, readily absorbed by carotene (red color); risk of thermal damage relatively low.
2.	Argon (CW or pulsed)	514 nm (blue-green)	Low absorption in H_2O and tooth. Absorption in hemoglobin. Risk of thermal damage relatively low.
3.	KTP laser (Kallium titanyl phosphate crystal frequency doubled Nd: YAG laser, pulsed)	532 nm (green)	Relatively low absorption in H_2O and tooth. High absorption in hemoglobin; medium penetration depth into dental hard tissue.
4.	He–Ne laser (CW)	632 nm (red)	Relatively low absorption in H_2O and tooth mineral; absorption in pigments and hemoglobin, deeper penetration depth into dental hard tissue.
5.	Nd: YAG laser (pulsed)	1064 nm (NIR)	Low absorption in H_2O and tooth; absorbed in dark pigments, deep penetration into dental hard tissue pulp damage due to temperature rise.
6.	Diode laser (CW or pulsed)	810, 830, 980 nm (NIR)	Low absorption in H_2O and tooth mineral, absorbed in pigments deep penetration into dental hard tissue – pulp damage due to temperature rise.
7.	Er, Cr: YSGG laser (pulsed)	2790 nm (SWIR)	Very high absorption in H_2O and tooth (OH^-). Low penetration depth into dental hard tissue, relatively low risk of direct pulp damage.
8.	Er: YAG laser (pulsed)	2940 nm (SWIR)	Highest absorption in H_2O and tooth. Low penetration depth into dental hard tissue, relatively low risks of pulp damage.
9.	CO_2 laser (CW/pulsed)	9400, 10600 nm (LWIR)	Highest absorption in H_2O and tooth (PO_4^-), low penetration depth into dental hard tissue, relatively low risk of pulp damage using pulsed mode.

which can be used are *KTP, He–Ne, diode and Er:YAG*. There are 2 ways to use lasers for bleaching—individually or in combination.[53]

How do Lasers Work on Bleaching Process?

Lasers are used to enhance the activation of bleaching materials. The lasers provide energy for hydrogen peroxide (H_2O_2) to breakdown into H_2O and O_2 and to release oxygen into the stained tooth. They catalyze the oxidation reaction. The free radicals of oxygen liberated in the process break apart the double valence bonds into simpler more stable less pigmented chains (Garber).[53]

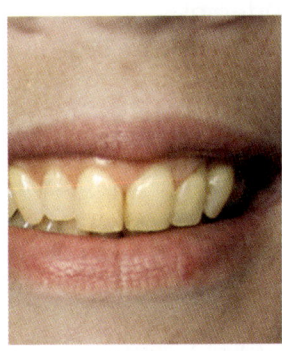 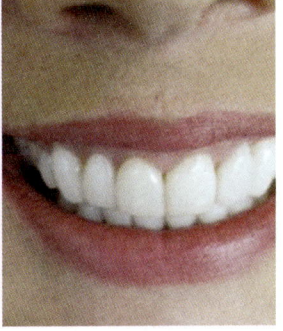

| Before | After |

Fig. 9.7

The expeditious rate reaction in laser bleaching has one major beneficial difference when compared with other methods of bleaching. Enough research has been concluded to assure clinicians that laser bleaching using argon laser as an energy source in the tooth-whitening process.[53] These two components, the ideal energy source and high concentration of the bleaching gel meet all the criteria required for achieving the ultimate rate of reaction. The bleaching process is a chemical reaction composed of different factors that determine the rate of the chemical reaction. The increase of the temperature, concentration of the reactants,

and intensity of the light in a photochemical reaction are all proportional to the rate of the chemical reaction of the tooth whitening.[53]

The pH value plays an important role in the rate of reaction in the bleaching process as well. Ionization of buffered hydrogen peroxide in the pH range of 9.5 to 10.8 produces more hydroxyl HO^{2-} free radicals. The result is a 50% greater bleaching effect in the same time as other pH levels. The average pH value found in various strengths of hydrogen peroxide is approximately 4.[53] The acidity allows the hydrogen peroxide to have a longer shelf-life; however, to achieve efficiency standards, it should be buffered to a much higher pH value with the salt of an alkaline base before being used as an agent for tooth whitening. A thickening agent is added for ease of control and handling.[53]

General Protocol of Laser Bleaching

Evaluate the dental condition: Review the patient's oral habit and health history, lifestyle, and expectations. Identify the type of stain and confirm the shade with the patient by using the Vita shade guide arranged by the value as:

B1/A1/B2/D2/A2/C1/D4/A3/D3/B3/ A3.5/B4/C3/A4/C4.

Discuss existing restoration and condition (limitations).

Take a photographic record (and study models for take-home bleaching trays).

Discuss possible treatment sensitivity and other treatment options.

Set-up: First-aid kit must contain anti-oxidants, such as vitamin E and aloe vera, and anti-inflammatory, such as zinc oxide and propylene glycol in addition to an eye wash bottle. Assemble protection gears like laser safety eye goggles, 2″ × 2″, 3 × 3″ gauze, cotton rolls, cheek retractor, and rubber dam. [53]

Preparation Kit[53]

- Plain pumice paste mixed with 3% hydrogen peroxide and rubber cup
- Floss, interproximal strips
- Brushes, water in a cup
- Etching gel (phosphoric acid 37.5%)
- Fluoride gel or rinse
- Extra-fine Soflex disks or Shofu polishing disks

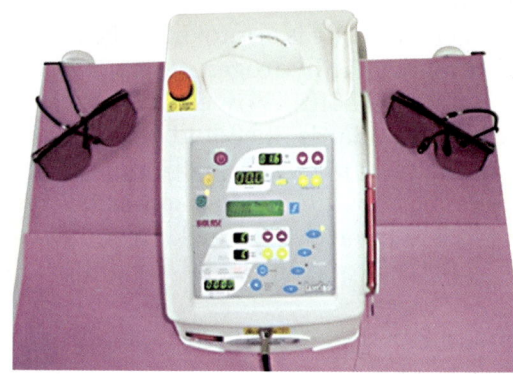

Fig. 9.8

Bleaching Kit

- 35 to 50% hydrogen peroxide bleaching gel or paste
- Brushes
- Mixing pad, spatula

Bleaching procedure[53]

1. Begin coronal cleansing with pumice.
2. Etch enamel for 5 to 1 second.
3. Wipe off, and rinse clean.
4. Perform isolation.
5. Brush the prepared bleaching medium carefully on the enamel area.
6. Activate laser light. Use the following settings: 0.35 W for 10-second duration for argon laser.
7. Expose each tooth for 10 seconds, and then repeat. Each tooth can receive 30 to 60 seconds lasing per application or until the color of the bleaching gel changes (blue to white; red to clear; yellow to clear).
8. Wipe off the used bleaching medium with wet gauze or cotton pellets or brush for interproximal area. Do not rinse with water.
9. Continue to paint on the fresh bleaching medium and activate until done.
10. Wipe off and repeat with the third application. When the third application is done, wipe off the gel, irrigate with water,
11. Remove isolation gear, and rinse well for 1 minute with fluoride rinse.
12. Polish the tooth surface with extra-fine polishing disks.

Additional Considerations

Consider covering bicuspid-to-bicuspid area, upper and lower arches. It varies in each individual situation; a single dark tooth or an unevenly colored area will need more applications.[53]

Have a team assistant hold another light unit, such as a plasma-arc lamp, to expose only 10 seconds per tooth. This speeds the process. Keep the bleaching compound 0.5 mm away from the gingival or root surface.[53]

Difficult cases (e.g. tetracycline stains) can take five applications, or schedule the patient for an additional bleaching appointment as well as continued treatment with the home bleaching method.[53] The combination of one visit of power bleaching and short-term home bleaching is an effective approach to tooth whitening. Larger teeth with thicker enamel respond more favorably with better results. Small teeth with thinner enamel have less bleaching effect with a higher chance of unfavorable pulpal response.[53]

Patients with prior bleaching experience respond to the laser bleaching quickly and favorably.

Advantages of Laser Bleaching

1. Laser bleaching is faster due to the high concentration of active ingredient (Christensen et al, 1997).[140]

2. It may act as a 'jump start ' for difficult cases by helping remove difficult stains caused by tetracycline and fluorosis.[140]

Disadvantages of Laser Bleaching [140]

1. High initial purchasing cost of the kit.

2. Time consuming procedure.

3. High postoperative sensitivity.

4. Anecdotal and empirical reports suggest moderate-to-severe post-procedural pain following laser-assisted bleaching (*ADA Council on Scientific Affairs 1998*).

Safety Issues in Laser Bleaching

There are no compromises when it comes to safety; responsible clinicians must recognize the operational parameters of the energy source selected. The argon-curing laser falls in the class III laser classification; this requires special training for operating the equipment and use of special eye protection with orange-colored lenses.[140] The eyes are sensitive photoreceptors; everyone in the operatory area must wear these glasses. The intensity of the light used for bleaching must be blocked out with glasses with the proper optical density for specific wavelengths.[140]

One must handle the caustic hydrogen peroxide with extreme caution. The patient should be acquainted fully with the procedure and well protected with a good isolation technique.[140] There are different techniques for isolating the bleaching site, such as the well-ligated traditional rubber dam, painting a gingival barrier, or merely working with lip and cheek retractors. A first-aid kit should contain antioxidants, such as vitamin E in liquid or capsule form and aloe vera gel. Even with all isolation techniques in place, a single spilled droplet of hydrogen peroxide or bleaching compound, within seconds, blanches and burns gingival tissue.[140] The patient may express discomfort with body language because the isolation techniques in place may make verbal communication impossible. The clinician should remain calm and apply the vitamin E oil quickly; the symptoms subside within 1 minute.[140]

The clinician must follow the protocol regarding the length of exposure time for the selected energy source, which depends on the intensity of the light (mW/cm²) and the particular wavelength.[140] The shorter the wavelength, the higher the energy of the photon. Conversely, longer wavelengths carry lower energy with more of the thermal effect of the photon. The general rule for avoiding unfavorable pulpal responses is 30 seconds per tooth because its thermal energy is at a higher energy output. Usually, there is a recommended time period for chemical oxidation followed by the light oxidation (5 minutes for argon laser and 10 minutes for plasma-arc lamp).[140]

10

Laser Safety

Safety is an integral part of providing dental treatment with a laser instrument. Lasers carry along with them a high risk of severe injury and damage.[50]

There are 3 facets to laser safety

1. Manufacturing process of the instrument
2. Proper operation of the device, and
3. The personal protection of surgical team and the patient

LASER HAZARD CLASSIFICATION

The intent of laser hazard classification is to provide working by users by identifying the hazards associated with the corresponding levels of accessible laser radiation through the use of labels and instructions. It also serves as a basis for defining control measures and medical surveillance.[50]

Laser and laser systems received from manufacturers are required by Federal law, 21 CFR Part 1000 to be classified and appropriately labeled by the manufacturer.[50]

Laser Hazard Classes

Laser and laser systems are assigned one to four broad classes (Class I to IV) depending on the potential of causing biological damage.[50]

• Provides a clear and concise indication that
  a laser system is in use
• Four signs available

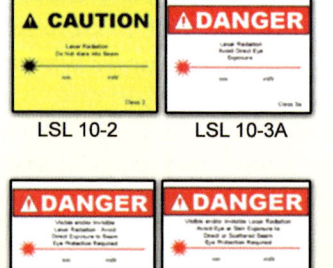

LSL 10-2   LSL 10-3A

LSL 10-3B   LSL 10-4

Related products

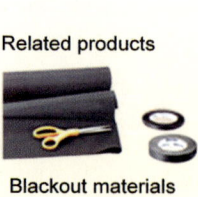

Blackout materials

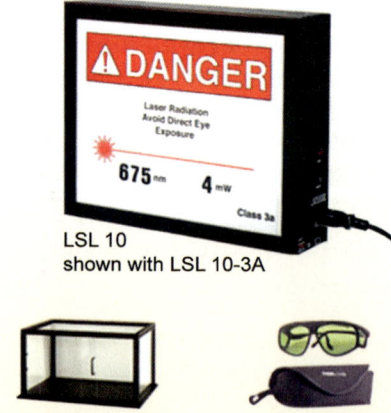

LSL 10
shown with LSL 10-3A

Enclosure systems   Safety googles

Fig. 10.1

122

The ANSI standard Z136.1 – 2000 documents set standards for classification in the U.S. OSHA and the American Conference of Government Industrial Hygienists also use this standard as a source.[50]

The classes are differentiated by a combination of output power of continuous emission laser or energy per pulse for pulsed lasers and the amount of time the beam is viewed.[50]

Class I

- Safe laser devices
- Do not pose a health hazard
- Totally enclosed, beam does not exit the housing

Condition: Below 40 (blue) and 100 mW in red spectral range.

Output power: Measured in one-tenth of a millimeter.

Examples: Laser caries detection systems, CD players.

Protective measures: None.

Warnings: None.

Remarks: Safe for naked eye but involve a safety hazard when using optical instruments, i.e. magnifying instruments (Also termed as *Class IM laser*).

Class I A

A special designation that is based on a 1000 second exposure and applies only to lasers that are *"not intended to viewing"*, such as supermarket laser scanner. The upper limit of Class IA laser is 4.0 mW. The emission of class IA laser is defined such that emission does not exceed the class I limit, e.g. of 1000 seconds.

Class II

- Emits only visible light.
- Low power output.
- Do not pose health hazard because of normal blinking and aversion reaction.

Condition: For CW lasers, output power has to below 1 mW.

Examples: Laser pointers, supermarket bar code scanner, laser caries detection.

Protective measures: None.

Warnings: Laser radiation. Do not stare into the beam.

IIa: Hazardous when viewed directly for more than 1000 seconds.

IIb: Dangerous as viewing time is one-fourth of a second, which is the time of an ordinary blinking reflex.

Class III A

- Intermediate power lasers.
- CW – 1 to 5 mW.
- If viewed momentarily, will not harm the unprotected eye.
- Have a caution label on them.

Class III B

- Moderate power laser

Output power: Continuous wave: 5–500 mW, pulsed: 10 J/cm^2.

Example: Argon curing laser, laser for measurements and shows, low-level lasers for therapeutic purposes.

Protective measures: Laser protective eyewear.

Warnings: Laser radiation. Avoid exposure to beam.

- In general, class IIIB lasers will not be a fire hazard, nor they generally capable of producing a hazardous diffuse reflection. Specific controls are recommended.
- According to new laser safety standard IEC 60825 – 1, this class is renamed as *"Class 3R"*.

Class IV

- High power lasers.
- Output power: 500 mW in CW or pulsed emission mode.

Class	UV	VIS	NIR	IR	Direct ocular	Diffuse ocular	Fire
I	X	X	X	X	–	No	No
IA	–	X°	–	–	Only after 1000 sec.	No	No
II	–	X	–	–	Only after 0.25 sec	No	No
III A	–	X°°	X	X	Yes	No	No
III B	X	X	X	X	Yes	Output is near Class IIIB limit	No
IV	X	X	X	X	Yes	Yes	No

Table 10.1: Summary of hazards

Key: X   = Indicates class applies in l range
       X° = Not intended for vowing only
       X°° = CDRH assigns class 3 B to visible l only

- Hazardous for direct viewing and may produce hazardous diffuse reflections.
- Also produces fire and skin hazards (Figs 10.2 and 10.3).

  Examples: Lasers for dental material processing, lasers for medical therapeutic users.

Protective Measures

- Technical protective measures for danger zone.
- Laser safety officer (LSO)
- User training
- Considerations for fire hazards.

  Warnings: Laser radiation, avoid skin/eye exposure to direct/scattered beam radiation.

NON-BEAM LASER HAZARDS

1. **Explosion hazards:** High-pressure arc lamps or filament lamps or laser welding equipment shall be enclosed in housings which can withstand maximum pressures. The laser target and elements of laser operation shall be enclosed.[50]
2. **Optical radiation hazards:** This relates to optical beam hazards other than laser beam hazards. UV radiation emitted from laser discharge tubes; pumping lamps and laser welding plasma shall be suitably shielded to reduce exposure levels.[50]

3. **Electrical hazards:** Corresponds to the method of electrical installation and connection to power supply circuit. All equipment shall be installed accordance with ANSI specifications 136.1 (1993).[50]

Summary of all the hazards is described in Table 10.1.

Biological Effects

1. Eye Injury

The eye is a critical target for laser injuries. The dentist, assistant, patients who are under a nominal hazard zone are at a risk from direct and reflected radiation of class III and IV Lasers.[50]

For example, cornea, which comprises some % of H_2O, absorbs the emission wavelengths of Er:YAG, CO_2 and Ho: YAG lasers which leads to corneal burn. The erbium and holomium lasers also affect the unprotected aqueous and vitreous humor and lens of eye, leading to aqueous flare and possibly contributing to *cataract formation*.[50]

Retinal damage occurs primarily with lasers that have more depth of penetration and are highly absorbed into pigment. These lasers have a shorter wavelength and include argon, He–Ne, diode and Nd:YAG. Retina is approximately 100,000 times more vulnerable to injury

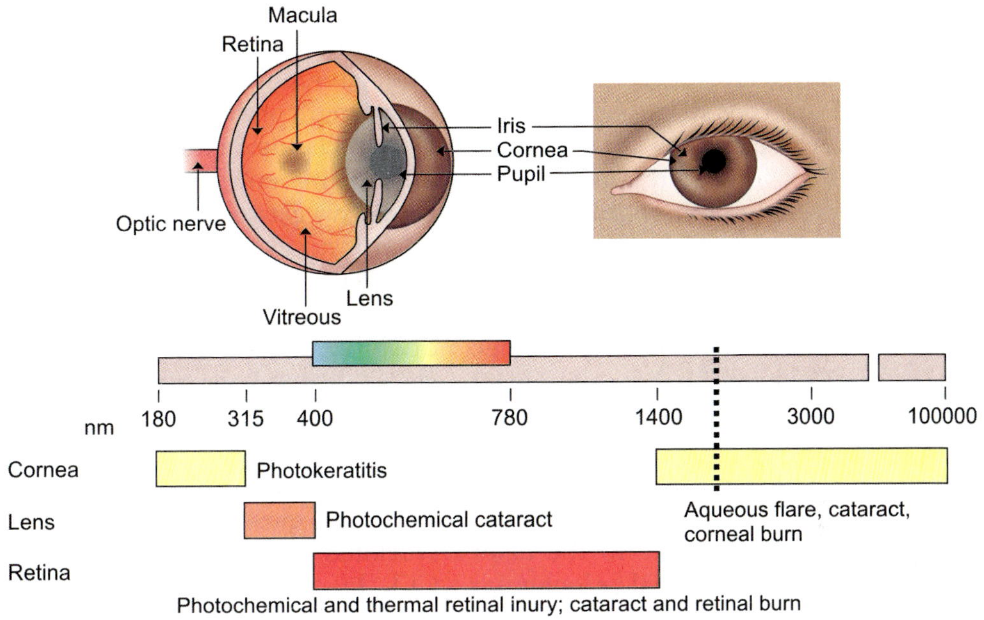

Macula
Retina
Iris
Cornea
Pupil
Optic nerve
Lens
Vitreous

| nm | 180 | 315 | 400 | | 780 | 1400 | | 3000 | 100000 |

Cornea — Photokeratitis

Lens — Photochemical cataract

Retina

Aqueous flare, cataract, corneal burn

Photochemical and thermal retinal inury; cataract and retinal burn

Fig. 10.2: Laser safety ocular hazards

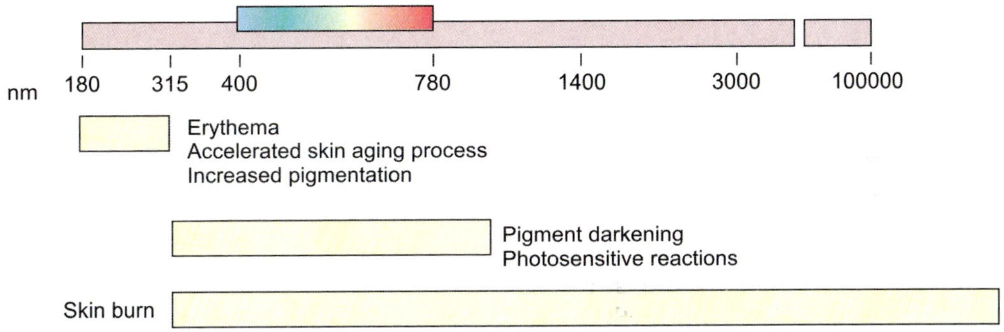

| nm | 180 | 315 | 400 | 780 | 1400 | 3000 | 100000 |

Erythema
Accelerated skin aging process
Increased pigmentation

Pigment darkening
Photosensitive reactions

Skin burn

Fig. 10.3: Laser safety skin hazards

than skin within retinal hazard range (l emission = 400 – 1400 nm). Laser-induced retinal damage results in irreversible loss of function.[50]

2. Others

Photochemical reactions are the principal causes of threshold level tissue damage following exposures to actinic ultraviolet radiation for any exposure time or "blue– light" visible radiation when exposures are greater than 10 seconds.[50]

Hyperpigmentations of skin and erythema are also caused by lasers of UV A and B range. Unprotected personnel may be exposed to extremely hazardous levels of beam power.[50]

SAFETY PROTOCOL

Development of an effective laser safety protocol that stresses compliance and meticulous attention to detail by the surgeon, and operating room nurse (laser surgery team) is probably the single most important reason this potentially dangerous surgical instrument can be used so safely in treating patients. Such a laser safety protocol is usually enough to list all the major and most minor precautions necessary when laser surgery is being performed. General considerations concern the provision for protection of the eyes and skin of patients and operating room personnel, as well as the provision for adequate laser plume (smoke) evacuation from the operative field. [50]

Eye protection: Depending on the wavelength, corneal or retinal burns, or both, are possible from acute exposure to the laser beam. The possibility for corneal or lenticular opacities (cataracts) or retinal injury exists following chronic exposure to excessive levels of laser radiation.[50] Several different structures of the eye are at risk; the area of injury usually depends on which structure absorbs the most radiant energy per volume of the tissue. Retinal effects occur when the laser emission wavelength occurs in the visible and near-infrared range of the electromagnetic spectrum (0.4 to 1.4 µm). When viewed either directly or secondary to reflection from a specular (mirror-like) instrument surface, laser radiation within this wavelength range would be focused to an extremely small spot on the retina, causing serious injury. This occurs because of the focusing effects of the cornea and the lens.[50]

Laser radiation in the ultraviolet region (less than 0.4 µm) or in infrared range of the spectrum (greater than 1.4 µm) produce effects primarily at the cornea, although certain wavelengths also may reach the lens. To reduce the risk of ocular damage during cases involving the laser, certain precautions should be followed. Protection of the eyes of the patient, surgeon and other operating room personnel must be addressed. The actual protective device will vary according to the wavelength of the laser used.[50] A sign should be placed outside the operating door warning all persons entering the room to wear the protective glasses because the laser is in use. In addition, extra glasses for the specific wavelength in use at the time should be placed on a table immediately outside the room. The doors to the operating room should remain closed during laser surgery with the CO_2 laser and locked when working with Nd:YAG or argon laser.[50]

All operating room personnel should wear protective glasses with side protectors. When working with operating microscope and the CO_2 laser, the surgeon need not wear protective glasses; here the optics of the microscope provides necessary protection (Ossiff et al, 1983). When working with the Nd:YAG laser, all operating room personnel must wear wavelength specific protective glasses that are usually of a blue-green color.[50] The patient's eyes should also be protected with a pair of these glasses. Though it may appear that the beam direction and point of impact are confined, inadvertent reflection of the beam may occur because of a faulty contact, or a break in the fiber. Special wavelength specific filters are available, when those filters are in place, the surgeon need not wear protective glasses.[50]

When working with the argon, KTP, or dye lasers, all personnel in the operating room, including the patient, should again wear wavelength-specific protective glasses, which are usually of an amber color. When performing photocoagulation procedures for the selected vascular lesions of the face, protective metal eyeshields rather than protective glasses are usually used on the patient. Similar precautions are necessary for newer visible and near infrared wavelength lasers. The major difference is the type of eye protection that is worn.[50]

Skin protection: A double layer of saline-saturated surgical towels, surgical sponges, or lap pads should protect all exposed skin and mucous membranes of the patient outside the surgical field. Great care must be exercised to keep the wet draping from drying out; it should be moistened from time to time during procedure. Teeth in the operating field also need to be protected. Saline saturated surgical sponges, or specially constructed metal dental impression trays can be used. Meticulous attention is paid to the protective draping procedures at the beginning of the surgery; the same compulsion should be displayed for the continued protection of the skin and teeth during the surgical procedure.[50]

Smoke evacuation (Fig. 10.4): Two separate suction set ups should be available for all laser cases. One provides for adequate smoke and steam evacuation from the operating field, while the second is connected to the surgical suction tip for the aspiration of blood and mucus from the operating field.[50] When performing laser surgery with closed anesthetic system, constant sectioning should be used to remove laser-induced smoke from the operating room. This helps to prevent inhalation by the patient, surgeon, or operating room personnel. A recent report has suggested that the smoke created by the interaction of the CO_2 laser with tissue is probably mutagenic (Tomita et al, 1981). Filters in the suction lines should be used to prevent clogging by the black carbonaceous smoke debris created by the laser.[50]

Instrument selection: The surface characteristics of instruments used in laser surgery should provide low specular or direct reflectance and large diffuse or scattered reflectance of the laser beam, should the beam inadvertently strike the instrument. Plastic instruments should be avoided since they can melt with the laser irradiation. Use of instruments with these characteristics will contribute to minimizing tissue injury from direct or reflected laser beam irradiation.[50]

Anesthetic considerations: Optimal anesthetic management of the patient undergoing laser surgery must include attention to the safety of the patient, the requirements of the surgeon, and the hazards of the equipment.[50]

Effectiveness of a safety protocol: Strong and Jako (1972) and later Snow et al (1976) warned of the possible complications associated with laser surgery (e.g. tissue damage) from reflection of the laser beam. Following these early warnings, several reports of complications uniquely attributable to use of CO_2 laser appeared in the literature.[50] In a survey of laser-related complications reported by Fried (1984) 49 of the 152 surgeons who used the laser reported 81 complications. Paper published by Ossoff on laser-related complications concluded that

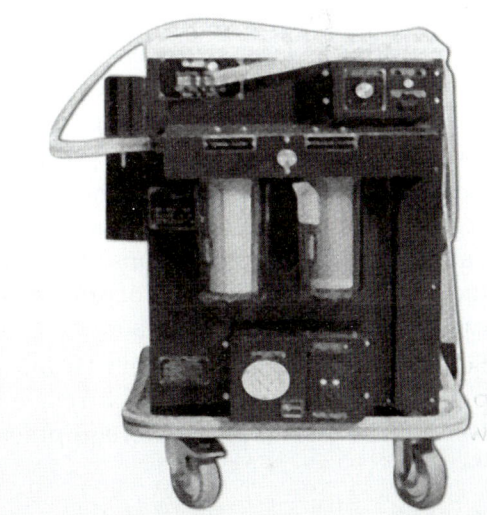

Fig. 10.4: Surgical laser smoke evacuator for removal of air-borne contaminants (laser plume) generated during laser surgery

certain precautions are necessary when performing laser surgery and, adherence to a rigid safety protocol allows laser surgery to be performed safely and with an extremely small risk of serious complications.[50]

LASER SAFETY OFFICER (LSO)

An LSO is a designated trained person who directs laser safety practices and ensures a safe environment while laser is in use. The *main task* of LSO is to support and advise the responsible operator concerning protective measures and safe operation of the laser device.[50]

Specific Tasks of LSO[50]

1. Hazard analysis in rooms where laser is operated comprising definition of danger zone.

2. Advising the responsible operator and supervisors of laser areas regarding safety aspects, purchasing and starting of laser devices and arrangements concerning occupational medicine.

3. Choice of personal protection equipment.

4. Cooperating in laser safety education for employees working with laser devices or in laser control area concerning hazards and protective measures.

5. Cooperating in examination and official acceptance of laser devices according to national rules and regulations. Assuring the maintenance and service of devices are carried out by qualified personnel.

6. Scheduled checks on observations of prescribed protection measures, e.g. wearing of personal protection equipment, installation of protective screens and warning signs, standardized methods and procedures for adjustment tasks.

7. Informing the responsible operator and supervisors of laser areas of defects in and failures of laser devices.

8. Investigation of all accidents and incidents in which laser were involved and forwarding of all relevant information on preventive actions including the safety officers.

Additional Tasks

1. Decisions on technical and operational protective measures.

2. Advising employees working with lasers or supervising them.

3. Stopping the use of lasers, if necessary.

4. Contacting authorities and keeping in touch with them.

How Safe are Dental Lasers?

Lasers are excellent tools, but carry along a high risk of injury and damage laser radiation mainly endangers eyes and skin. Hence, these risks warrant suitable protective measures with their strict observation being the responsibility of employer and management.[50]

Impact of laser radiation on biological tissue not only depends on radiation parameters (e.g. wavelength intensity or irradiation time), but also on irradiated tissue.

Thus, when it comes to laser safety, there should be no compromises and then, lasers in dentistry will offer incredible precision, less pain, faster healing and of course safety.[50]

11

The Future of Lasers in Dentistry

Laser technology is developing very quickly. New lasers with a wide range of characteristics are available today and are being used in the various fields of dentistry. The search for new devices and technologies for dental procedures was always challenging and in the last two decades much experience and knowledge has been gained.

Clinical lasers are of two types: Soft lasers are essentially an aid to healing with relatively few rigorous studies available to support their use. Surgical *hard lasers*, however, can cut both hard and soft tissues and replace the scalpel and drill in many areas. From initial experiments, with the ruby laser, most clinicians are using argon, CO_2 and now Nd:YAG systems. The first dental laser based on an Nd:YAG engine provides handpieces of similar size to conventional instrumentation and being fed by a fiberoptic 'cable', has the flexibility for intraoral use that the CO_2 lasers, widely used in oral surgery. Furthermore, extensive clinical investigation has demonstrated their safety in clinical practice and the fact that procedures can usually be performed without a local anesthetic is obviously seen as a considerable advantage by patients. Sterilizing as it cuts, the Nd:YAG laser promises to find uses not only in caries removal and soft tissue surgery but also in endodontics and gingival curettage.

Lasers will have a definitive place in dentistry in the future but to be practical, one dental laser will have to be applicable to a number of therapeutic procedures. Due to its very favorable absorption on dental hard tissues, the CO_2 laser will also undoubtedly be useful for many other procedures in dental practice. A long-needed characteristic of a laser has been the simultaneous delivery or blending of several wavelengths in the range of CO_2, argon and Nd:YAG lasers that would offer the advantage of both cutting and coagulation. With free electron laser, this application is theoretically possible using one machine with the same optical system. The availability of new wavelength will also lead to the development of dyes less toxic than the ones now available.

After Maiman's invention of the ruby laser, researchers were able to create lasing with other solid-state substances as well as gases and liquids. Although research laboratories around the world have experimented with the entire chart of the electromagnetic spectrum for lasing capabilities, certain wavelengths have become the standard for dental applications.

The first of these wavelengths to be cleared to market by the US Food and Drug Administration (FDA) for intraoral use was the carbon dioxide (CO_2) laser. The real interest for the use of lasers in dentistry occurred in the early 1990s with the introduction of the pulsed neodymium: yttrium-aluminum-garnet (Nd:YAG) laser which was followed shortly thereafter by the argon and various erbium (Er) and diode wavelengths. As of this writing, the three best markets for dental lasers have been Germany, Japan, and the United States. Of total world sales, the United States' market represents 40 to 50%; Japan 30 to 35%; and Germany 20 to 25%.

Future Advances in Laser Technology

Many dentists may use size and pricing as excuses for not purchasing lasers. Most dentists do have a space problem or a concern that prices are still too high. The last 10 years have seen a sometimes-significant reduction in size and price of dental lasers.

Size: The trend in smaller sizes will continue in the future to the point of shrinking most lasers to small tabletop or hand-held instruments. The US military already has fabricated a hand-held laser coagulator for field use. The active medium used in this small military laser is specific configuration of semi-conducting wafers (diode bars). It is diode technology, either used as the active medium itself or as a pumping mechanism to drive other solid-state lasers that will help make future lasers more efficient and much smaller.

Presently, dental diode lasers are commercially available in either 800 to 830 nm or 950 to 1010 nm wavelengths. This number will increase in the future; medical diodes are presently available in six different wavelengths. Diode lasers are efficient converting 30% of input electric power into laser output power. This can be compared with about 1 to 2% electric efficiency for most lamp-pumped solid-state lasers. Thus was born the idea of replacing flash-lamps with appropriate wavelengths of diode lasers and creating diode-pumped solid-state lasers. Because they are more efficient than their flash-lamp-pumped counterparts, require smaller power supplies and cooling mechanisms and can be manufactured at a reduced size and cost.

Another benefit of using diode lasers to pump solid-state lasers is that possibility of using new and different active media that presently cannot be stimulated by flash or arc lamps, creating totally new laser wavelengths. Diode technology advancements will play a major role in the future of lasers in dentistry.

Price: It is a simple concept, prices decrease and sales increase. Price will decrease over time for three reasons:
- Increased use of diode technology
- Increased sales
- Competition

In addition to the obvious psychological benefit, lower pricing would have on the dental market, the real advantage is that more lasers would be sold. As annual revenues increase, new markets could be developed overseas, which would increase sales and revenues further. This cycle is important for the future of lasers in dentistry because without increased revenues, manufacturers cannot fund research and development properly.

Several FDA clearances accruing in the late 1990s sparked a renewal of interest within the dental community, and accordingly a notable increase in laser sales was noted. The trend may continue for the next several years, if not decades. The dental market has the ability to lead the way for increased expenditures in research and development, which, in turn, can develop more efficient lasers, discover new active media and delivery systems, and control prices.

Advances in Laser Dentistry

It has been said that the laser is an invention in search of an application. That was true in dentistry during the 1990s. When the first Nd:YAG dental laser appeared in the US market, claims were made for a myriad of applications concerning both hard and soft dental tissues. As more wavelengths appeared, more claims followed. It did not take long to discover that some of the stated claims were inaccurate or unsubstantiated (or both). Thanks to a tremendous amount of research, training, and education, clinicians now know which laser to use and when. But what about the future? What can dentists look forward to the first couple of decades of the twenty-first century?

Replacing the high-speed turbine: Ultimately, laser technology will replace the air turbine for composite restorations, G.V. Black preparations, full crowns, inlays, onlays, finish lines, and old restorations. Scanning electron microscopic images of human enamel with various geometric shapes drilled into its surface showed to have sharp line and point angles, and their walls were parallel to one another. The instrument used to cut these shapes was a pulsed neodymium: yttrium-lanthanum-fluoride (Nd: YLF) laser (1053 nm).

Caries inhibition: In 1980, Yamamoto and Katsuhiko reported that Nd:YAG lasing could prevent dental caries in enamel. Although Powell's group has investigated caries inhibition with the argon laser, Featherstone's work with the CO_2 laser has shown the most promise in the area of research. To date, all of Featherstone's investigations had been in vitro studies. Featherstone believes, however, that clinical studies could begin within 2- to 3-year period (personal communication, February 1997) and that within the next 10 to 15 years a small inexpensive CO_2 laser designed specifically for caries inhibition will be used by the hygienist as part of the standard treatment for caries prevention

Curing: During the 1990s, composite restorative materials have gained popularity. Their increased usage caused researchers to develop small, low-power argon lasers (488 nm) for curing composites. With the advances being made in diode technology, within the next 5 years a small hand-held blue diode laser will replace all current curing systems.

Detecting caries: An alternative to using radiographs in dentistry may be an imaging technique known as terahertz pulsing imaging. Terahertz waves or millimeter waves are located just below the infrared band in the electromagnetic spectrum and are generated by lasing semiconductors with ultrafast pulses (femtoseconds) of visible laser light. Although terahertz pulse imaging research is still in an early stage, researchers presently can shift contrast mechanisms to measure specific thickness or tooth enamel, peer inside the dentin for caries, or construct a movable three-dimensional image of the tooth on a computer screen. A different system being developed at the University of Strathclyde's Institute of Photonics in Glasgow, Scotland, uses a diode-pumped chromium: lithium-sulphur-argon-flourine (Cr:LiSAF) laser (850 nm) to take advantage of the tooth's natural ability to fluorine. The technology differs from the argon laser's ability to excite fluorophors because in contrast to the argon, this unit can penetrate and give readings of the enamel greater than 0.5 mm deep.

Optical coherence tomography (OCT) is another technology that may replace dental radiographs. Optical coherence tomography is similar to ultrasound but uses light waves instead of acoustic waves to interact with the target tissue to create images. In contrast to ultrasound, optical coherence tomography does not require a conducting medium. Although all three systems are a few years from being seen in any dental office, they have major advantages over current X-ray technology in that they do not use ionizing radiation and are much more sensitive in recording changes in demineralization of the tooth. In the future, one of these technologies plus the use of the CO_2 caries inhibition laser are to be powerful tools in caries management.

Selective caries and calculus removal: To date, at least two wavelengths have capabilities to ablate selectively specific components of teeth, while not affecting adjacent tooth structures. The free-running pulsed Nd:YAG laser can remove enamel caries yet has virtually no effect on caries-free enamel whereas the frequency-doubled alexandrite laser can remove calculus from root structure and not harm the surrounding cementum. Although both of these procedures have clinical significance, because of its cost factor the alexandrite laser may never be seen in the market place, if more clinical applications cannot be found for this laser. The reason is purely economic in nature.

Endodontics: In the early 1990s, xenon chloride excimer laser was used to clean and shape the root canal, eliminating the need for files and reamers.

The goal of researchers and manufacturers has to be to identify a wavelength that would replace reamers and files, have other hard or soft tissue applications, are cost-effective, and are at least as effective as conventional root canal therapy. Although there has been a large amount of research in laser endodontics using various wavelengths, no system has been built to meet all the previously stated requirements. Even though many German dentists are using the free-running pulsed Nd:YAG and diode lasers for adjunctive root canal therapy, as of this writing, only a handful of lasers have FDA clearance in the United States. That clearance limits the laser's use only to coronal pulp procedures; however, change is expected.

Once the needed FDA clearance for total laser endodontics is obtained, the unit will probably be an infrared wavelength, and its delivery system will be use a small (50 to 200 µm) optic fiber that will have the ability to side-fire. It is predicted that gutta-percha will be replaced with flowable composite material that will be injected into the lased canal and cured with the small hand-held blue diode laser. A system as just described would save valuable clinical time by eliminating the shaping of the canal that is presently necessary to accommodate the gutta-percha cones. Most of the aforementioned components exist today; their safety and effectiveness need to be demonstrated.

Cosmetic dentistry: Practically, every dentist lecturing on cosmetic dentistry and advocates the use of lasers to shape or contour the oral soft tissue because of:

1. Less bleeding,
2. Better visualization of treatment site,
3. No post-surgical tissue shrinkage,
4. Decrease in post-surgical discomfort,
5. The ability to make final impressions on the same day as laser surgery, and
6. Decreased need for injections.

As lasers continue to be recommended for soft tissue manipulation, laser cosmetic surgery will become standard of care within the next 10 years. Lasers are better and have unique advantages for the patient and clinician over steel blades or electro-surgery.

Another area that is seen and becoming more diversified in usage is computer-aided design/computer-aided manufacturing (CAD/CAM) systems which use lasers for measuring the internal and external shapes of the tooth. For the dentist using this technology in the office, the systems not only will have the capability of fabricating single units (inlays, onlays, and crowns) more precisely than with casting technology, but also preparing multiple fixed units. In the future, dental laboratories will use CAD/CAM technology to fabricate the framework for fixed or removable prostheses. (Presently, dental laboratories use special Nd:YAG lasers for welding purposes because of their advantages over conventional welding techniques).

Low-level laser therapy: Low-level laser therapy (LLLT) is based on the concept that certain low-level doses of specific coherent wavelengths can turn on or off certain cellular components or functions. Practically speaking, dentists outside the United States (no FDA clearance yet for such devices) have been administering LLLT to their patients as an aid in healing, reducing pain and swelling, and controlling oral infections for at least the past 3 decades. The research shows that LLLT works, but out of the thousands of studies that exist using LLLT, few represent good evidence-based research. The lasers that are used most commonly are the helium-neon (633 nm) or diode (820 or 940 nm) with power outputs well below 1W.

In 2008, a laser-related trade journal printed an article on dental laser indicating that because of new applications, reduced prices, and instruments becoming more user-friendly, the dental laser market in the US was becoming a billion dollar industry. If the same has to hold true in India, keeping in mind the huge dental market, several criteria must be met:

- Market penetration must be double in the next 4 to 5 years.
- Instrument sizes must diminish.
- Laser prices must decrease.

Meeting these criteria would generate the necessary revenues for increased expenditures for research and development to improve existing delivery systems and develop fiber types, continue development of a short-pulsed hard tissue laser to replace air turbines, and combine wavelengths into a single package, while looking into new wavelengths. If all of the above-mentioned become a reality in 10 to 15 years, the growth of the dental laser market could be limitless because of the worldwide dental marketplace. The last 20 years have witnessed many new developments in dental technologies, and the next 20 years promise to be even richer in technologic advancements. *Lasers will be in the forefront of that growth.*

12

Before Purchasing a Dental Laser

Before buying a laser, clinicians should attend national meetings where lasers are being presented and also attend an introductory laser course. As long as you assess the variety of devices in the marketplace, commit to attending standard proficiency dental laser certification as recognized by the academy of laser dentistry, and proceed through the learning curve at a pace comfortable for you, the rewards will be noticed quickly by your staff, patients, and practice.

First Things First

Before you purchase a dental laser, consider your type of practice and learn about the different laser wavelengths and their recommended applications. Matching the laser wavelength to your practice needs is important. What this really means is that you begin your laser education prior to making a purchasing decision.

Sorting through Marketing Hype

There are many manufacturer-based training courses, and the old adage "let the buyer beware" applies. It is important to understand basic laser physics, laser safety, clinical uses, different laser wavelengths, power settings, and various tissue interaction effects. Attend an introductory course. A general introduction to laser technology includes most laser devices currently available in the marketplace.

With the assistance of corporate member manufacturers who willingly provide devices for introductory courses, the side-by-side evaluation provides access to and understanding of lasers in a nonselling environment. Make your purchasing decision based on sound scientific evidence and your own particular needs—not upon the misconception that lasers will revolutionize your dental practice.

Questions to Ask

- What features do I want or need?
- What procedures have been cleared for marketing by the US Food and Drug Administration?
- What procedures do I currently perform that can be assisted with laser technology?
- What procedures do I not perform that I would consider providing for my patients if I had a laser?
- How much training and certification do I need?
- What are the regulatory issues, if any, in my state dental practice act?
- How do I successfully incorporate laser technology into my practice?

- What technical support is available, and is it consistent?
- How long has the device been on the market, and what is the company's track record for efficiency, reliability, and serviceability?

LASER DEVICE CHECKLIST

- *Range of applications, speed of performance, precision, and controllability:* Currently, there are 23 indications for laser use cleared for marketing by the FDA. No single laser can perform all applications equally well under all conditions. Lasers should be a part of the conventional armamentarium. In some cases, it can be the primary instrument of choice; in others, it can be an adjunctive instrument.

- *Delivery systems, ease of use, disposable components:* The laser's delivery system is one of the most important considerations. Does the delivery system provide intraoral accessibility to your satisfaction? How easily are components changed in the middle of a procedure for the desired tissue interaction?

- *Design limitations, safety, sterilization, and infection control:* Is the laser designed specifically for dental use? What are the power requirements and external cooling system requirements (if any)? What are the built-in safety features? How easy is it to sterilize and disinfect the laser, the individual components, and accessories?

- *Cost (initial, maintenance, and replacements):* The range of laser purchase prices may be anywhere from $6,700 to $78,000 (soft and hard tissues) depending upon numerous features, delivery systems, wavelengths, and add-on components. Consider the cost over the expected lifetime of the device, not just the initial purchase. As with any well-managed practice implementation, consider the learning curve for you as a practitioner and for your staff.

- *Ease of set up, use, and portability; control panel displays; foot pedals:* Is the laser easy to set up in your operatory? Can you easily transport the laser between operatories? Is the control panel easily viewable? Are power settings pre-set, and how easy is it to change those settings as needed? Is the activation of the foot pedal easily accessed? Is the pedal adequately protected from inadvertent activation? Are power settings preset? Can you easily adjust those settings?

- *Quality of construction, beam alignment, and calibration; upgradeability:* Is calibration of the device easily achieved? How often, if ever, is calibration necessary? Does the design of the laser lend itself to upgrade capability, if appropriate? Does the manufacturer support such a program?

- *Features and accessories:* Learn about the accessories that may require separate purchases. Consider cost and ease of replacement. Assess the features and accessories relative to your clinical setting.

- *Manuals, training, troubleshooting:* Do training manuals include indications for use, suggested power settings for particular procedures, and methods to adjust any factory presets? Is manufacturer training provided, and how is it provided—in your office or in a seminar setting?

- *Track record, warranty, and service:* Ask hard questions about customer satisfaction and talk with actual dentist customers. What is the track record of the manufacturer or distributor? How responsive are they? If factory-serviced, consider how the device is to be repackaged for shipment and whether the manufacturer provides shipping support. Compare warranties. Determine how often you should reasonably expect to use the warranty provisions and how quickly issues are resolved.

INTERNATIONAL ORGANIZATIONS DEDICATED TO USE OF LASERS

1. Academy of Laser Dentistry (ALD): *www.laserdentistry.org*
2. American society for Laser Medicine and surgery: *www.aslms.org*
3. Society for Oral Laser Applications : *www.sola-int.org*
4. Laser Institute of America: *www.laserinstitute.org*
5. SPIE : *www.spie.org*
6. World Association for Laser Therapy: *www.walt.nu*
7. World Federation for Laser Dentistry: *www.wfld-org.info*

NATIONAL ORGANIZATIONS DEDICATED TO USE OF LASERS

A. Indian Academy of Laser Dentistry (iald.co.in)

1. Post-graduate advanced certificate course–laser dentistry—6 months
2. Diploma in laser dentistry—6 months
3. Diploma in diode laser dentistry—3 months
4. Introduction to laser dentistry—2 days

B. Society of Oral Laser Application (solaindia.org)

1. Diploma in laser dentistry—10 days in india
2. Masters in laser dentistry—in Vienna

C. L.D.D.R.—Academy for Laser Dentistry Education (ldrr.org)

1. Basic course in laser dentistry—2 days

D. Sri Sai College of Dental Surgery (sscds.edu.in)

1. Certificate course in laser dentistry—6 months

E. Dr. Jamuna Pai's Institute of Medical and Aesthetic Cosmetology (djpimac.com)

1. Basic course in lasers and light devices in esthetic practice—1 month

F. Chennai Dental Research Foundation (chennaidentalresearch.com)

1. Laser dentistry course—270 working days

Before Purchasing

- Examine your practice needs, wants, and goals.
- Attend a dental laser introductory course and ask questions.
- Compare devices and arrange for in-office demonstrations.
- Talk with other laser users.
- Critically evaluate the available information.

After Purchasing

- Obtain training for the device from the manufacturer.
- Attend a standard proficiency dental laser certification course that includes lecture, hands-on, written examination, and clinical simulation examinations.
- Start slowly and realize there is a learning curve. Keep it simple and increase your confidence over time.
- Realize that dental laser education is continual.

Leading Laser Manufacturers

- BIOLASE Technology (www.biolase.com)
- DEKA Laser Technology (www.dekalasers.com)
- Hoya ConBio (www.conbio.com)
- Incisive (www.incisivelaser.com)
- Ivoclar Vivadent (www.ivoclarvivadent.us.com)
- KaVo America (www.kavousa.com)
- Lares Research (www.laresdental.com)
- Lumenis (www.lumenis.com)
- Millennium Dental Technologies (www. millenniumdental.com)
- Sirona (www.sirona.com)
- Syneron (www.syneron.com)
- Zap Lasers (www.zaplasers.com)

Glossary

Ablation: The removal of material in industrial laser cutting, or tissue in medical laser cutting, by melting, evaporation, or vaporization.

Absorb: To transform radiant energy into a different form, with a resultant rise in temperature.

Absorption: Transformation of radiant energy to a different form of energy by the interaction of matter, depending on temperature and wavelength.

Absorption coefficient factor: Describes light's ability to be absorbed per unit of path length.

Active medium: Collection of atoms or molecules which can be stimulated to a population inversion, and emit electromagnetic radiation in a stimulated emission.

Afocal: Literally, "without a focal length"; an optical system with its object and image point at infinity.

Aiming beam: A laser (or other light source) used as a guide light. Used coaxially with infrared or other invisible light, may also be a reduced level of the actual laser used for surgery or for other applications.

Absorption coefficient: A measurement of the amount of absorption of laser energy, expressed as a relative number per unit area.

Active medium: The material within the optical cavity that, when stimulated and amplified into a population inversion, will emit laser energy. This medium may be an ion, molecule, crystal, semi-conductor wafer, or combination of gases. A synonymous term is lasant.

Amplification: A process that occurs within the optical resonator whereby stimulated emission produces a population inversion.

Articulated arm: A laser delivery system that uses segments of a hollow tube that are coupled with right angle mirrors that allows propagation of the laser beam along its length.

Attenuation: The observed decline in energy as a beam passes through an absorbing or scattering medium.

Average power: An expression of the average of the peak power and the laser off time.

Amplification: The process in which the electro-magnetic radiation inside the active medium within.

Amplitude: The maximum value of the electro-magnetic wave measured from the mean to the extreme; simply stated: the height of the wave.

Accessible emission level: The magnitude of accessible laser (or collateral) radiation of a specific wavelength or emission duration at a particular point as measured by appropriate methods and devices. Also means radiation to which human access is possible in accordance with the definitions of the laser's hazard classification.

Accessible emission limit (AEL): The maximum accessible emission level permitted within a particular class. In ANSI Z 136.1, AEL is determined as the product of accessible emission maximum permissible exposure (MPE) limit and the area of the limiting aperture (7 mm for visible and near-infrared lasers).

Attenuation: The decrease in energy (or power) as a beam passes through an absorbing or scattering medium.

Argon laser: A gas laser in which argon ions are the active medium. This laser emits in the blue-green visible spectrum, primarily at 488 and 515 nm.

Axis/optical axis: The optical centerline for a lens system; the line passing through the center of curvature of the optical surfaces of a lens.

B

Beam: A collection of rays that may be parallel, convergent, or divergent.

Beam diameter: The distance between diametrically opposed points in the cross-section of a circular beam where the intensity is reduced by a factor of e-1 (0.368) of the peak level (for safety standards). The value is normally chosen at e-2 (0.135) of the peak level for manufacturing specifications.

Beam divergence: Angle of beam spread measured in radians or milliradians (1 milliradian = 3.4 minutes of arc). For small angles where the cord is approximately equal to the arc, the beam divergence can be closely approximated by the ratio of the cord length (beam diameter) divided by the distance (range) from the laser aperture.

Beam spot size: The diameter of the laser beam which can vary with the focal distance.

Beam splitter: An optical device used to divide the light from a laser into two separate beams—the reference beam and the object beam. It consists of a partially transparent mirror that reflects part of the laser beam and transmits the rest.

C

Carbon dioxide (CO_2) laser: A gas laser in which CO_2 molecules are the active medium. This laser emits in the infrared spectrum, with the strongest emission line at 10.6 µm. It can be operated in either CW or pulsed mode.

Cathode: The negative electrode of a gas laser used for electrical excitation of the gas in the tube.

Chromophore: A light-absorbing compound or molecule normally occurring in tissues that is an attractor of specific wavelengths of laser energy.

Coherence: A term describing light as waves which are in phase in both time and space. Monochromaticity and low divergence are two properties of coherent light.

Coherency: A term that describes all of the radiant waves traveling in phase both temporally and spatially.

Collimated light: Light rays that are parallel. Collimated light is emitted by many lasers. Diverging light may be collimated by a lens or other device.

Collimation: Ability of the laser beam to not spread significantly (low divergence) with distance.

Cladding: A thin coating that surrounds the core of glass in a fiberoptic delivery system. The cladding maintains the propagation of the laser beam along the glass. The cladding is surrounded by a thicker jacket to aid in flexibility.

Coagulation: An observed denaturation of soft tissue proteins that occurs at 60°C.

Contact mode: The direct touching of the laser delivery system to the target tissue.

Continuous mode: The duration of laser exposure is controlled by the user (by foot or hand switch).

Continuous mode: A manner of applying laser energy in which beam power density remains constant over time; also termed continuous wave and abbreviated CW.

D

Delivery system: The manner in which laser energy is transferred to the target tissue. For dental lasers, there are fiberoptic, hollow waveguide, and articulated arm systems. Some of these systems employ additional tips.

Diffraction: The bending of a light ray as the light passes through a medium; also known as refraction.

Divergence: An observed degree of spread of the laser beam as it increases its distance from the emission aperture or focal point; the opposite of collimation.

Diode laser: A laser whose active medium consists of an array of semiconductor wafers, pumped with electrical current, whose beams are collected and focused into a beam. The emission wavelengths can range from the visible into the near-infrared thermal portion of the electromagnetic spectrum.

Diode: An electronic device that conducts a current in only one direction.

Dosimetry: Measurement of the power, energy, irradiance, or radiant exposure of light delivered to tissue.

Doping: The addition of an element to the laser crystal, resulting in a specific emission of energy. An example is doping an yttrium aluminum garnet crystal with the element of erbium.

Duty: Cycle ratio of total "on" duration to total exposure duration for a repetitively pulsed laser.

E

Electromagnetic radiation: Flow of energy consisting of oscillating electric and magnetic fields lying transverse to the direction of the wave's propagation.

Electromagnetic spectrum: A graphic representation of all forms of radiant energy from gamma rays to radio waves and usually depicted with increasing wavelength and/or decreasing frequency.

Energy (Q): The capacity for doing work. Energy is commonly used to express the output from pulsed lasers and it is generally measured in Joules (J). The product of power (watts) and duration (seconds). One watt second = one Joule.

Energy density: The measurement of energy per unit area, usually expressed as joules/square centimeter; also known as fluence.

Embedded laser: A laser with an assigned class number higher than the inherent capability of the laser system in which it is incorporated, where the system's lower classification is appropriate to the engineering features limiting accessible emission.

Emission: Act of giving off radiant energy by an atom or molecule.

Enclosed laser device: Any laser or laser system located within an enclosure which does not permit hazardous optical radiation emission from the enclosure. The laser inside is termed an "embedded laser".

Enhanced pulsing: Electronic modulation of a laser beam to produce high peak power at the initial stage of the pulse. This allows rapid vaporization of the material without heating the surrounding area. Such pulses are many times the peak power of the CW mode (also called "Superpulse").

Excimer laser: A gas laser which emits in the UV spectrum. The active medium is an "Excited Dimer" which does not have a stable ground state.

Excitation: Energizing the active medium to a state of population inversion.

Excited state: Atom with an electron in a higher energy level than it normally occupies.

Erbium: A rare earth element that is used to dope a crystal of yttrium aluminum garnet or yttrium scandium gallium garnet.

Excited state: An atom or molecule with electron orbit(s) in an energized or higher level than the resting state.

External power source: An energy system outside the laser's optical resonator that provides for the excitation and stimulation of the active medium; also known as a pumping mechanism.

F

Fiberoptic: A delivery system composed of a glass fiber which may be stranded and is used to propagate the laser beam along its length. The glass is surrounded by cladding and a jacket or layers of jackets.

Fluence: See energy density.

Focal length: The distance between the focusing lens and the focal point, which is the place where the laser beam's power and energy are delivered at maximum value. It is usually measured in millimeters. In bare fiberoptically delivered lasers, the focal length is essentially zero, since the greatest emission is at the end of the fiber, used in contact with the tissue. In other delivery systems, such as an articulated arm, the focal point is usually several millimeters from the end of the delivery system.

Focal point: That distance from the focusing lens where the laser beam has the smallest diameter.

Free-running pulse mode: A laser operating mode where the emission is truly pulsed and not gated. A flashlamp is used as the external energy source so that very short pulse durations and peak powers of thousands of watts are possible. A laser operating in this mode cannot be operated in continuous wave.

Frequency: The number of oscillations or cycles of a wave, usually expressed per second.

G

Gas laser: A laser in which the active medium is a gas. The gas can be composed of molecules (e.g. CO_2), atoms (e.g. He–Ne) or ions (e.g. Ar^+).

Gated pulse mode: A laser operating mode where the emission is a repetitive on and off cycle. The laser beam is actually emitted continuously, but a mechanical shutter or electronic controls 'chop' the laser beam into pulses. This term is synonymous with chopped pulse mode.

Gaussian curve: A graphic depiction of normal distribution of an entity. For lasers, it illustrates the cross-section of the power density during a certain time period, usually a pulse.

H

Handpiece: An instrument attached to the distal portion of the delivery system that contains the focusing lens system. In some cases, an additional tip is attached to the handpiece to complete the assembly.

Helium–neon (He–Ne) laser: A laser in which the active medium is a mixture of helium and neon. Its wavelength is usually in the visible range. Used widely for alignment, recording, printing, and measuring.

Hertz: For lasers, the number of pulses per second, repetition rate, or pulse rate. Unfortunately frequency can also be expressed in hertz, but that terminology is not used in laser discussions.

Hollow wave guide: A delivery system that uses a flexible hollow tube with a mirrored inner surface to propagate the laser beam along its length.

I

Incident light: A ray of light that falls on the surface of a lens or any other object. The "angle of incidence" is the angle made by the ray with a perpendicular (normal) to the surface.

Infrared radiation (IR): Invisible electromagnetic radiation with wavelengths which lie within the range of wavelength from 700 nm to 1 mm. This region is often broken up into IR-A, IR-B, and IR-C.

Infrared spectrum (IR): Invisible electromagnetic radiation between 0.7–1,000 [μm].

Ion laser: A laser in which the active medium is composed of ions of a nobel gas (gas such as argon or krypton). The gas is usually excited by high discharge voltage at the ends of a small bore tube.

Ionizing radiation: Radiation commonly associated with X-ray or other high energy electromagnetic radiation which will cause DNA damage with no direct, immediate thermal effect. Contrasts with non-ionizing radiation of lasers.

Intensity: The magnitude of radiant energy.

Irradiance (E): Radiant flux (radiant power) per unit area incident upon a given surface. Units: Watts per square centimeter.

J

Joule (J): A unit of energy (1 watt-second) used to describe the rate of energy delivery. It is equal to 1 watt-second or 0.239 calorie. A basic unit of energy.

K

KTP (Potassium titanyl phosphate): A crystal used to change the wavelength of an Nd:YAG laser from 1060 nm (infrared) to 532 nm (green).

L

Laser: An acronym for light amplification by stimulated emission of radiation. A laser is a cavity with mirrors at the ends, filled with material, such as crystal, glass, liquid, gas or dye. It produces an intense beam of light with the unique properties of coherency, collimation, and monochromaticity.

Laser medium (active medium): Material used to emit the laser light and for which the laser is named.

Laser pulse: A discontinuous burst of laser radiation, as opposed to a continuous beam. A true laser pulse achieves higher peak powers than that attainable in a CW output.

Laser rod: A solid-state, rod-shaped lasing medium in which ion excitation is caused by a source of intense light, such as a flash lamp. Various materials are used for the rod, the earliest of which was synthetic ruby crystal.

Laser system: An assembly of electrical, mechanical and optical components which includes a laser. Under the Federal Standard, a laser in combination with its power supply (energy source).

Laser safety officer (LSO): One who has authority to monitor and enforce measures to the control of laser hazards, and effect the knowledgeable evaluation and control of laser hazards.

Lens: A curved piece of optically transparent material which depending on its shape is used to either converge or diverge light.

Lenses: Lenses are devices that redirect light. In photography, lenses are used to focus an image for the film. Holographers use lenses to widen a laser's beam to illuminate the entire object being holographed.

Light: Usually refers to the visible spectrum. The range of electromagnetic radiation frequencies detected by the eye, or the wavelength range from about 400 to 700 nm. The term is sometimes used loosely to include radiation beyond visible spectrum limits.

M

Maximum permissible exposure (MPE): The level of laser radiation to which person may be exposed without hazardous effect or adverse biological changes in the eye or skin.

Meter: A unit of measurement and for electromagnetic waves used to describe the wavelength. For dental lasers, it is divided by a million and termed a micron or micrometer; or divided by a billion and termed a nanometer.

Micrometer: A unit of length in the International System of Units (SI) equal to one millionth of a meter. Often referred to as a "micron".

Micron: An abbreviated expression for micrometer which is the unit of length equal to 1 millionth of a meter (10^{-6} [m]).

Monochromatic: The characteristic of a laser beam where only one wavelength is present.

Mode: A term used to describe how the power of a laser beam is geometrically distributed across the cross-section of the beam. Also used to describe the operating mode of a laser, such as continuous or pulsed.

N

Nanometer (nm): A unit of length in the International System of Units (SI) equal to one billionth of a meter. It is the usual measure of light wavelength. Visible light ranges from about 400 nm in the purple to about 700 nm in the deep red.

Nanosecond: One billionth of a second. Longer than a picosecond or femtosecond, but shorter than a microsecond. Associated with Q-switched lasers.

Nd:Glass laser: A solid-state laser of neodymium glass offering high power in short pulses in which a Nd doped glass rod is used as a laser active medium, to produce 1064 nm wavelength.

Nd:YAG laser: A solid-state laser in which neodymium-doped yttrium aluminum garnet is used as a laser active medium, to produce 1064 nm wavelength. YAG is a synthetic crystal.

Neodymium (Nd): The rare earth element that is the active element in Nd:YAG and Nd:Glass lasers.

Nominal hazard zone (NHZ): The nominal hazard zone describes the space within which the level of the direct, reflected, or scattered radiation during normal operation exceeds the applicable MPE. Exposure levels beyond the boundary of the NHZ are below the appropriate MPE level.

Nominal ocular hazard distance (NOHD): The axial beam distance from the laser where the exposure or irradiance falls below the applicable exposure limit.

Non-contact mode: The delivery system is used without touching the target tissue.

O

Output coupler: The part of the laser which enables light to come out of the laser. Usually, it is a partially reflecting mirror at the end of the laser optical cavity.

Optical fiber: A filament of quartz or other optical material capable of transmitting light along its length by multiple internal reflection and emitting it at the end.

Optical pumping: The excitation of the active medium in a laser by the application of light, rather than electrical discharge. Light can be from a conventional source, like xenon or krypton lamp, or from another laser.

Output power: The energy per second (measured in watts) emitted from the laser in the form of coherent light.

Optical resonator (optical cavity): The component of a laser containing the active medium in which the population inversion occurs. At each end of the resonator, there are reflective surfaces or mirrors which produce amplification and coherency. The distal mirror is partially transmissive; when there is sufficient energy, the beam can exit through that mirror.

P

Peak power: The measurement of power in each pulse.

Photon: A unit or quantum of radiant energy.

Plume: Essentially, the smoke produced as by products due to the laser-tissue interaction. It is composed of particulate matter, cellular debris, carbonaceous and inorganic materials, and potentially bio-hazardous products.

Population inversion: A state within the laser cavity in which the quantity of excited species of the active medium exceeds that of the unexcited species (those at the resting, stable state.)

Power: The amount of work performed per unit time, expressed in Watts.

Power density: The measurement of power per unit area, usually expressed as Watts/square centimeter; also known as intensity, irradiance, and radiance.

Pulse duration: A measurement of the total amount of time that the pulse is emitted; also known as pulse width.

Pulse frequency: The rate at which pulses are generated. Pulse frequency is expressed in pulses per second (Hz).

Pulse: A discontinuous burst of laser, light or energy, as opposed to a continuous beam. A true pulse achieves higher peak powers than that attainable in a CW output.

Pulsed laser: A laser which delivers energy in the form of a single pulse, or train, of laser pulses.

Pumping: The process of applying energy to the active medium from an external energy source.

Q

Q-Switch: A device that produces very short (~ 10–250 ns), intense laser pulses by enhancing the storage and dumping of electronic energy in and out of the lasing medium.

Q-Switched laser: A laser which store energy in the active medium, to produce short pulse with high energy. It is done by blocking the resonator ability to oscillate, keeping the "Q-Factor" of the optical cavity low.

R

Radiant energy (Q): Energy in the form of electromagnetic waves usually expressed in units of Joules (watt-seconds).

Radiant energy: Laser energy emitted expressed in joules (J).

Radiant exposure (H): The total energy per unit area incident upon a given surface. It is used to express exposure to pulsed laser radiation in units of J/cm^2.

Radiant power: Laser power emitted expressed in watts (W).

Reflection: The returning of electromagnetic radiation by surfaces upon which it is incident. The two general

types are specular, which is created from a smooth polished surface; and diffuse, which emanates from a rough surface.

Refraction: The change of direction of propagation of any wave, such as an electromagnetic wave, when it passes from one medium to another in which the wave velocity is different. The bending of incident rays as they pass from one medium to another (e.g. air to glass).

Resonator: The mirrors (or reflectors) making up the laser cavity including the laser rod or tube. The mirrors reflect light back and forth to build up amplification.

Retina: The sensory tissue that receives the incident image formed by the cornea and lens of the human eye. The retina lines the posterior eye.

Ruby laser: The first laser type; a crystal of sapphire (aluminum oxide) containing trace amounts of chromium oxide as an active medium.

S

Selective photothermolysis: A precise laser tissue interaction in which the radiation is well absorbed and the pulse duration is shorter than the thermal relaxation time which minimizes tissue damage.

Semiconductor laser: A type of laser which produces its output from semiconductor materials, such as gallium arsenide (GaAs).

Solid state laser: A laser in which the active medium is in solid state (usually not including semiconductor lasers).

Source: The term "source" means either laser or laser-illuminated reflecting surface, i.e. source of light.

Spontaneous emission: The release of energy (a photon) as the previously excited particle level returns to its resting, stable state.

Stimulated emission: The release of energy (a photon) from an already excited particle by interaction with a particle of identical energy, producing two coherent particles. This process was theorized by Albert Einstein in 1916 and is the basis for laser operation.

Spot size: The mathematical measurement of the radius of the laser beam.

Superpulse: Electronic pulsing of the laser-driving circuit to produce a pulsed output (250–1000 times per second), with peak powers per pulse higher than the maximum attainable in the continuous wave mode. Average powers of superpulsed lasers are always lower than the maximum in continuous wave. Process often used on CO_2 surgical lasers.

A variation of gated pulsed mode in which the pulse durations are very short, producing high peak power; also termed very short pulse.

T

TEA laser: An acronym for transversely excited atmospheric laser. This CO_2 gas laser uses a transverse flow of gas and operates at higher pressures than other gas lasers, generally near atmospheric pressure. The result is a higher energy beam.

Thermal effect: For lasers, the absorption of the radiant energy by tissue producing an increase in temperature.

Thermal relaxation time: The amount of time required for temperature of the tissue that was raised by absorbed laser radiation to cool down to one-half of that value immediately after the laser pulse.

Transmission: The passage of electromagnetic radiation through any medium.

TEM (Transverse electromagnetic modes): Used to designate the cross-sectional shape of the beam. The radial distribution of intensity across a beam as it exits the optical cavity.

TEM00: The lowest order transverse mode possible. The power distribution across the beam is of a bell-shaped (Gaussian) shape.

Tunable dye laser: A laser whose active medium is a liquid dye, pumped by another laser or flash lamps, to produce various colors of light. The color of light may be tuned by adjusting optical tuning elements and/or changing the dye used.

Tunable laser: A laser system that can be "tuned" to emit laser light over a continuous range of wavelengths or frequencies.

U

Ultraviolet (UV) radiation: Electromagnetic radiation with wavelengths between soft X-rays and visible violet light, often broken down into UV-A (315–400 nm), UV-B (280–315 nm) and UV-C (100–280 nm).

V

Vaporization: The physical process of converting a solid or liquid into a gas; for dental procedures, it describes conversion of liquid water into steam.

Visible radiation: Light-electromagnetic radiation which can be detected by the human eye. It is commonly used to describe wavelengths which lie in the range between 400 nm and 700 nm. The peak of the human spectral response is about 555 nm.

W

Watt: An expression of power.

Watt/cm²: A unit of irradiance used in measuring the amount of power per area of absorbing surface, or per area of CW laser beam.

Wavelength: The distance between any two similar points on a wave; for example, from peak to peak, measured in meters.

Y

YAG: An acronym describing a solid crystal of yttrium-aluminum-garnet that can be doped with various rare earth elements and is used as an active medium for some lasers.

YSGG: An acronym describing a sold crystal of yttrium, scandium, gallium and garnet that can be doped with various rare earth elements and is used as an active medium for some lasers.

References

1. Hussein A. Applications of lasers in dentistry: A review. *Archives of Orofacial Sciences 2006;1:1–4.*

2. Sonju Clasen AB, Ogaard B, Duschner H, Ruben J, Arends J, Sonju T, et al. Caries development in fluoridated and non-fluoridated deciduous and permanent enamel in situ examined by micro radiography and confocal laser scanning microscopy. *Adv Dent Res 1997;11(4):442–47.*

3. Hall A, Girkin JM. A review of potential new diagnostic modalities for caries lesions. *J Dent Res 83C; 2004:89–94.*

4. Hall A, Stookey GK. In vitro studies of laser fluorescence for detection and quantification of mineral loss from dental caries. *Adv Dent Res 1997;4:507–14.*

5. Knezevic A, Demoli N. Composite photo-polymerization with diode laser. *Operative Dentistry 2007;32(3):279–84.*

6. Knezevic A, Demoli N. Measurement of linear contraction using digital laser interferometry. *Operative Dentistry 2005;30(3):346–52.*

7. Knezevic A, Nazif Demoli, Zrinka Tarle. Digital Holographic Interferometry— A New method for measuring polymerization shrinkage of composite materials. *Acta Stomatol Croat 2005;39:155–60.*

8. Lussi A, Hack A, Hug I, et al. Detection of approximal caries with a new laser fluo-rescence device. *Caries Res 2006;40:97–103.*

9. Lussi A, Hibst R. DIAGNOdent: An optical method for caries detection. *J Dent Res 2004; C83:80–83.*

10. Ko ACT, Lin-Ping, Choo-Smith, Mark Hewko, Michael G. Sowa. Detection of early dental caries using polarized Raman spectroscopy. *Optics Express 2006;14(1):114–20.*

11. Moritz A, Schoop U. Procedures for enamel and dentin conditioning: a comparison of conventional and innovative methods. *Journal of Esthetic dentistry 1998;10(2) 84–93.*

12. Moritz A, Andriana da Costa Ribeiro. Effects of Diode laser (810 nm) irradiation on root canal walls: thermographic and morphological studies. *J Endod 2007;33:252–55.*

13. Ana Raquel Bennetti, Eduardo Batista Franco, Eric Jacomino, Jose Carlos Pereira. Laser therapy for dentin hypersensitivity: a critical appraisal. *J Oral Laser Application 2004;4: 271–78.*

14. Oza A. Dental and bone ablation. *J Endod 2007; 55(23):1–18.*

15. Rode A, Gamaly EG, B Luther Davies, et al. Precision ablation of dental enamel using a subpicosecond pulsed laser. *Australian Dental Journal 2003;48(4):233–239.*

16. Sønju Clasen A, Ruyter IE. Quantitative determination of type A and type B carbonate in human deciduous and permanent enamel by means of fourier transform infrared spectrometry. *Adv Dent Res 1997;11(4):523–27.*

17. Angmar-Mansson B, Ten Bosch JJ. Advances in methods for diagnosing coronal caries – a review. *Adv Dent Res 1993;7(2):70–79.*

18. Angmar-Mansson B, Ten Bosch JJ. Optical methods for the detection and quantification of caries. *Adv Dent Res 1987;1(1):14–20.*

19. Angmar-Mansson B, ten Bosch JJ. Quantitative light-induced fluorescence (QLF): a method for assessment of incipient caries lesions. *Dentomaxillofacial Radiology 2001;30:298–307.*

20. Goodman BD, Kaufman HW. Effects of an argon laser on the crystalline properties and rate of dissolution in acid of tooth enamel in the presence of sodium fluoride. *J Dent Res 1977;56(10):1201–07.*

21. Colston BW, Sathyam US, Da Silva LB, Everett MJ. Dental OCT. *Optics Express 1998;3(6): 230–38.*

22. Apel C, Duschner H, Meister J, et al. Structural changes in human dental enamel after sub ablative erbium laser irradiation and its potential use for caries prevention. *Caries Res 2005;39:65–70.*

23. Camila Pinelli, Monica Campos Serra, Leonor de Castro Monteiro Loffredo. Validity and reproducibility of a laser fluorescence system for detecting the activity of white spot lesions on free smooth surfaces in vivo. *Caries Res 2002; 36:19–24.*

24. Todea CDM. Laser applications in conservative dentistry. *TMJ 2004;54(4):392–402.*

25. Carmen Todea, Cristini Kerezi, Cosmin Balabuc, Mircea Calniceanu, Laura Filip. Pulp capping—from conventional to laser assisted therapy. *J Oral Laser Application 2008;8:71–82.*

26. Cozean C, Arcoria CJ, Pelagalli J, et al. Dentistry for the 21st century—Erbium: YAG laser for teeth. *J Am Dent Assoc 1997;128: 1080–87.*

27. Goya C, Matsumoto K, Yamazaki R, et al. Effects of pulsed Nd:YAG laser irradiation on smear layer at the apical stop and apical leakage after obturation. *International Endodontic Journal 2000;33: 266–71.*

28. Chia-Ling Tsai, Yng-Tzer Lin, Shun-Te Huang, et al. In vitro acid resistance of CO_2 and Nd:YAG laser-treated human tooth enamel. *Caries Res 2002;36:423–29.*

29. Buhler CM, Patara Ngaotheppitak, Daniel Fried. Imaging of occlusal dental caries (decay) with near-IR light at 1310-nm. *Optics Express 2005;13(2):573–82.*

30. Hsu CYS, Jordan TH, Dederich DN, et al. Laser-matrix-fluoride effects on enamel demineralization. *J Dent Res 2001; 80(9): 1791–801.*

31. Darling CL, Daniel Fried. Real-time near IR (1310 nm) imaging of CO_2 laser ablation of enamel. *Optics Express 2008;16(4):2685–93.*

32. Daniel Fried, Breunig T. Hard tissue ablation and modification with IR lasers. *J Biomedical Opt 2001;3:196–203.*

33. Daniel Fried, Breunig TS. Infrared spectroscopy of laser irradiated dental hard tissues using the advanced light source. *SPIE 2000;3910: 136–48.*

34. Daniel Fried, John DB, Featherstone. Early caries imaging and monitoring with near infrared light. *Dent Clin N Am 2005;49:771–93.*

35. Toscano DD, Hanriete Pereira de Souza. Study of human dentary tissues by laser-induced breakdown spectroscopy. *Applied Surface Science 1998(2):662–67.*

36. Harris DM, Daniel Fried. Pulsed Nd:YAG laser selective ablation of surface enamel caries: Photo acoustic response and FTIR spectroscopy. *SPIE BIOS 2000;3910–25.*

37. David A. Crawley, Christopher Longbottom, Cole BE, et al. Terahertz pulse imaging: A pilot study for potential applications in dentistry. *Caries Res 2003;37:352–59.*

38. Smith DL, Burnett AP, Thomas E. Gordon Jr. Laser welding of gold alloys. *J Dent Res 1972; 51(1):161–67.*

39. Don Arnone, Craig Ciesla. Terahertz imaging comes into view. *Physics world 2001.* Available from: www.eleceng.adelaide.edu.au/**thz**/documents/arnone_2001_pwo.pdf.

40. Coluzzi DJ. Fundamentals of dental lasers: science and instruments. *Dent Clin N Am 2004;48(4):751–68.*

41. Dederich DN, Buschick RD. Lasers in dentistry-separating science from hype. *JADA 2004; 135:204–11.*

42. Dederich DN. CO_2 laser fusion of vertical root fracture. *JADA 1999;130:1195–99.*

43. Park DS, Lee HJ, Yoo HM, Oh TS. Effect of Nd:YAG laser irradiation on the apical leakage

of obturated root canals: an electrochemical study. *International Endodontic Journal* 2001;34:318–21.

44. Viducic D, Jukic S, Karlovic Z, et al. Removal of gutta-percha form root canals using Nd:YAG laser. *International Endodontic Journal* 2003;36:670–73.

45. Fogleman EA, Kelly MT, Grubbs WT. Laser interferometric method for measuring linear polymerization shrinkage in light-cured dental restoratives. *Dental Materials* 2002;18:324–30.

46. Emin Esen, Oguz Yoldas. Apical microleakage of root end cavities prepared by CO_2 laser. *Journal of Endodontics* 2004;30(9):662–64.

47. Emma Pickwell, Wallace VP, Cole BE, et al. A comparison of terahertz pulsed imaging with transmission Microradiography for depth measurement of Enamel demineralization in vitro. *Caries Res* 2007;41:49–55.

48. Fabiola Galbiatti, Mario Alexandre Coelho. Confocal laser scanning microscopic analysis of the depth of dentin caries like lesions in primary and permanent teeth. *Braz Dent J* 2008; 19(2):139–44.

49. Feldchtein FI, Gelikonov GV. In vivo OCT imaging of hard and soft tissue of the oral cavity. *Optics Express* 1998;3(6):239–50.

50. Franziska Beer, Martin Strabl, Wernisch J. Laser safety. *J Oral Laser Applications* 2005; 5(2):71–79.

51. Margolis FS. Clinical uses of erbium laser. Available from: www.fredmargolis.com/ErbiumLasers.pdf

52. Gaetan Duplain, Russel Boulay, Belanger PA. Complex index of refraction of dental enamel at CO_2 laser wavelengths. *Applied Optics* 1987; 26(20):4447–51.

53. Freedman GA, Gerald McLauglin, Linda Green Wall. Power bleaching and in office techniques. In: Martin Dunitz (ed). *Bleaching Techniques in Restorative Dentistry*, 1st edition, 2002:140–42.

54. Stookey GK. Quantitative light fluorescence: a technology for early monitoring of the caries process. *Dent Clin N Am* 2005;49:753–70.

55. Stookey GK, Carlos González-Cabeza. Emerging Methods of caries diagnosis. *Journal of Dental Education* 2001;65(10):1001–6.

56. Giovanni Olivi, Maria Daniela Genovese. Erbium Chromium laser in pulp capping treatment. *J Oral Laser Applications* 2006;6: 291–99.

57. Glenn van As. Erbium lasers in dentistry. *Dent Clin North Am* 2004;48:1017–59.

58. Lynn Powell G, Patrick Kelsey W, Richard J. The use of argon laser for polymerization of composite resin. *Journal of Esthetic Dentistry* 1989;3:34–35.

59. Grace Sun. Role of Lasers in Cosmetic Dentistry. *Dent Clin North Am* 2000;44(4): 831–45.

60. Grace Sun, Jan Tuner. Low-level laser therapy in dentistry. *Dent Clin North Am* 2004; 48(4): 1061–76.

61. Heinz Duschner, Hermann Gotz, Roger Walker, et al. Erosion of dental enamel visualised by confocal laser scanning microscopy. In: Martin Dunitz (ed). *Clinical Advances in Restorative Dentistry*, 1st edition, 2000;67–73.

62. Tsuda H, Arends J. Orientational micro-Raman spectroscopy on hydroxyapatite single crystals and human enamel crystallites. *J Dent Res* 1994;73(11):1703–10.

63. Tsuda H, Arends J. Raman Spectroscopy in Dental Research: a short review of recent studies. *Adv Dent Res* 1997;111(4):539–47.

64. Pretty IA, Gerardo Maupomé, A closer look at diagnosis in clinical dental practice: Part 5- emerging technologies for caries detection and Diagnosis. *J Can Dent Assoc* 2004;70(8): 540–9.

65. Igor Cernavin, Hogan SP. The effects of Nd:YAG laser on amalgam dental restorative material. *Australian Dental Journal* 1999:44:2: 98–102.

66. Isao Ishikawa, Akira Aoki, Recent advances in surgical technology, *Ch.70 Peridontology, Carranza*, 1035–38.

67. Isauremi Vieira de Pinheiro, Maria Ângela Fernandez. Use of laser fluorescence (DIAGNODent) for in vivo diagnosis of occlusal caries: a systematic review. *J Appl Oral Sci* 2004;12(3):177–81.

68. Jack Hadley, Young DA, Eversole LR, et al. A laser-powered hydrokinetic system for caries

removal and cavity preparation. *J Am Dent Assoc 2000;131:777–85.*

69. Wallace JA. Effect of Waterlase laser retrograde root-end cavity preparation on the integrity of root apices of extracted teeth as demonstrated by light microscopy. *Aust Endod J 2006;32: 35–39.*

70. Janez Diaci. Laser profilometry for the characterization of craters produced in Hard dental tissues by Er:YAG and Er, Cr:YSGG Lasers. *Journal of the Laser and Health Academy 2008;1(2):1–10.*

71. Jenny Zachrisson, Occlusal caries detection and quantification with laser as a diagnostic tool, *Dept. of Cariology 1998;175–84.*

72. Beltrano JJ, Torrisi L. Er, Cr:YSGG pulsed laser applied to medical dentistry. *Radiation Effects and Defects in Solids 2008;163(4–6):331–38.*

73. Ten Bosch JJ. General aspects of optical methods in dentistry. *Adv Dent Res 1987;1 (1):5–7.*

74. Joel M White, Edward J Swift. Lasers for use in dentistry. *Journal of Esthetic and Restorative Dentistry 1991;11:455–61.*

75. John D. Preston, Reisbick M H. Laser fusion of selected dental casting alloys. *J Dent Res 1975;54(2):232–38.*

76. John D Featherstone, Nelson DGA. Laser effects on dental hard tissues. *Adv Dent Res 1987;1:21–26.*

77. John D. Featherstone B. The science and practice of caries prevention. *J Am Dent Assoc 2000;131:887–99.*

78. Vlacic J, Meyers IA, Walsh LJ. Laser-activated fluoride treatment of enamel as prevention against erosion. *Australian Dental Journal 2007;52:3:175–80.*

79. Kamburoglu, Barenboim SF. Quantitative measurements obtained by micro-computed tomography and confocal laser scanning microscopy. *Dentomaxillofacial Radiology 2008;37:385–91.*

80. Karen M McNally, Barrie RD Gillings, Judith M Dawes. Dye-assisted diode laser ablation of carious enamel and dentine. *Australian Dental Journal 1999;44(3):169–75.*

81. Koba K, Kimura Y, Matsumoto K, et al. A histopathological study of the morphological changes at the apical seat and in the periapical region after irradiation with a pulsed Nd:YAG laser. *International Endodontic Journal 1998;31: 415–20.*

82. Koshira K, Inoue S, Niimi K, et al Bond strength and SEM observation of CO_2 laser irradiated dentin, bonded with simplified step adhesives. *Operative Dentistry 2005;30(2):170–79.*

83. Koukichi Matsumoto. Laser treatment of hard tissue lesions. *J Oral Laser Applications 2004; 4:235–48.*

84. Koukichi Matsumoto, Yuichi Kimura. Laser therapy of dentin hypersensitivity. *J Oral Laser Application 2007;7:7–25.*

85. Walsh LJ. Pulpal temperature changes during low power hard tissue laser procedures, *Braz Dent J 1996;7(1):5–11.*

86. Walsh LJ. The current status of laser applications in dentistry. *Australian Dental Journal 2003;48(3):146–55.*

87. Walsh LJ. The current status of low level laser therapy in dentistry. Part 1. Soft tissue applications. *Australian Dental Journal 1997;42(4):247–54.*

88. Walsh LJ. The current status of low level laser therapy in dentistry. Part 2. Hard tissue applications. *Australian Dental Journal 1997;42(5):302–06.*

89. Walsh LJ. Laser analgesia with pulsed infrared lasers: theory and practise. *J Oral Laser Application 2008;8:7–16.*

90. Walsh LJ. Low level laser therapy. Available from:www.aegislasertherapy.com/Conditions/Dental1.pdf.

91. Bergmans L, Moisiadis P, Teughels W, et al. Bactericidal effect of Nd:YAG laser irradiation on some endodontic pathogens ex vivo. *International Endodontic Journal 2006;39:547–57.*

92. Ceballos L, Toledano M, Osorio R, Tay FR, Marshall GW. Bonding to Er:YAG-laser treated dentin. *J Dent Res 2002;81:2:119–22.*

93. Lena Nicolaides, Chris Feng, Andreas Mandelis, et al. Dental dynamic diagnostics using simultaneous frequency-domain PTR and Laser Luminescence. *Analytical Sciences 2001;17:331–33.*

148   Lasers in Operative Dentistry and Endodontics

94. Otis LL. Optical Coherence tomography: A new imaging technology for dentistry. *JADA* 2000;131:511–15.

95. Luciana Chucre, Sebastião Luiz. Clinical evaluation of dentin hypersensitivity treatment with low intensity gallium-aluminium-arsenide laser—GaAlAs. *J Appl Oral Sci* 2004; 12(4):267–72.

96. Mario Bertolotti. And finally the laser. In: Tom Spicer (ed). *The History of the Laser*, 7th edition, Bristol, The institute of physics publishing, 2005;245–78.

97. Fleming MG, Maillet WA. Photo polymerization of composite resin—using the argon laser. *Journal of Canadian Dental Association* 1999;65(8):447–50.

98. Miyazaki M, Moore BK. Analysis of dentin resin interface by use of Raman spectroscopy. *Dental Materials* 2002;18:576–80.

99. Nambiar KR, Lasers—principles, types and applications. In: Nambiar KR (ed). *Textbook of Lasers—Principles, Types and Applications*, 1st edition. New Delhi, New Age International Publishers 2004;3–12.

100. Claxton NS, Fellers TJ, Michael W Davidson. Laser scanning confocal microscopy. Available from citeseerx.ist.psu.edu/viewdoc/download?doi=10.1.1.113.8660

101. Ota Samek, Telle HH, Beddows DCS. Laser-induced breakdown spectroscopy: a tool for real-time, in vitro and in vivo identification of carious teeth. *BMC Oral Health* 2001;1:1.

102. Pallav Diamond G, Hutchins D, Gan TH. A near infrared technique for non-destructive evaluation. *Insight* 2008;50:5–10.

103. Patricia Moreira de FREITAS, Debora SOARES-GERALDO. Intrapulpal temperature variation during Er, Cr:YSGG enamel irradiation on caries prevention. *J Appl Oral Sci* 2008;16(2):95–9.

104. Photon-induced photo, acoustic streaming: the 1st real breakthrough, *Lares research and Fotona.* Available from: www.laresdental.com/downloads/files/PIPS_brochure.pdf.

105. Radmila Obradovic, Lijiljana Kesic, Ana Pejèiæ. Low level laser therapy of dentin hypersensitivity: a review. *Medicine and Biology* 2007;14(1):15–18.

106. Raj Wadhwani. Lasers in dentistry—An introduction to new technology. *International Dentistry SA* 2005;2:6–20.

107. Stern RH, Sognnaes RF. Lased Enamel: Ultra-structural Observations of pulsed carbon dioxide laser effects. *J Dent Res* 1972;51(2):455–60.

108. Lobene RR, Samuel Fine. Interaction of carbon dioxide laser radiation with enamel and dentin. *J Dent Res* 1968; 47(2):311–17.

109. Slusher RE. Laser technology. *Reviews of Modern Physics* 1999;71(2):71–9.

110. Jeon RJ, Han C, Mandelis A, Sanchez V, Abrams SH. Diagnosis of pit and fissure caries using frequency-domain infrared photo thermal radiometry and modulated laser luminescence. *Caries Res* 2004;38:497–513.

111. Jeon RJ, Mandelis A, Matvienko A, et al. Interproximal dental caries detection using photothermal radiometry (PTR) and modulated luminescence (LUM). *Eur Phys J Special Topics* 2008;153:467–69.

112. Conssivar RA. The biologic rationale for use of lasers in dentistry. *Dent Clin N Am* 2004; 48:833–60.

113. Strauss RA. Esthetics and laser surgery.

114. Jones RS, Gigi D Huynh, Graham C Jones, et al. Near-infrared transillumination at 1310 nm for the imaging of early dental decay. *Optics Express* 2003;11(18): 2259–65.

115. Robin Orchadson, David G Gillam. Managing dentin hypersensitivity. *JADA* 2006;137:990–96.

116. Rudiger Emshoff, Ivano Moschen. Use of laser Doppler flowmetry to predict vitality of luxated or avulsed permanent teeth. *Oral Surg Oral Med Oral Pathol Radiol Endod* 2004; 98:750–55.

117. Faller RV, Duschner H. Application of confocal laser scanning microscopy for studying remineralization and demineralization process. *ADA/FDI World Dental Congress* 1996;1–2.

118. Samraj RV, Indira R, Srinivasan MR, et al Recent advances in pulp vitality testing. *Endodontology* 2003;15:14–19.

119. Al-Khateeb S, Angmar-Månsson B, Ten Cate JM. Light-induced fluorescence studies on

dehydration of incipient enamel lesions. *Caries Res* 2002;36:25–30.

120. Al-Khateeb S, Ten Cate JM, Angmaar-Mansson B. Quantification of formation and remineralization of artificial enamel lesions with a new portable fluorescence device. *Adv Dent Res* 1997;11(4):502–06.

121. Jukic S, Anic I, Koba K, Matsumoto K. The effect of pulpotomy using CO_2 and Nd:YAG lasers on dental pulp tissue. *International Endodontic Journal* 1997;30:175–80.

122. Sofia Tranaeus, Angmar-Mansson B. In vivo repeatability and reproducibility of the quantitative light induced fluorescence method. *Caries Res* 2002;36:3–9.

123. Parker S. Introduction, history of lasers and laser light production. *British Dental Journal* 2007;202(1): 21–31.

124. Mesaros SV, Trope M. Revascularization of traumatized teeth assessed by laser Doppler flowmetry: case report. *Endod Dent Traumatol* 1997;13:24–30.

125. Tatjana Dostalova, Helena Jelinkova. Diode laser-activated bleaching. *Braz Dent J 15(Special issue)* 2004;S1-3–S1-8.

126. Thais Marcondes de Oliveira, Hanriete Pereira de Souza. Analysis of carious and non carious human dentin by laser-induced breakdown spectroscopy. *Applied Surface Science 1998; 127:662–67.*

127. Thereza Christina Pinheiro, Antonio Pinheiro. Laser treatment in the treatment of dentin hypersensitivity. *Braz Dent J 2004;15(2):144–50.*

128. Adams TC, Pang PK, Lasers in aesthetic dentistry. *Dent Clin N Am 2004;48:833–60.*

129. Timothy Frederick Watson. Fact and artefact in confocal microscopy. *Adv Dent Res 1997; 11(4):433–41.*

130. Timothy Frederick Watson, Boyde A. Operative dentistry and the abuse of dental hard tissues: Confocal microscopical imaging of cutting. *Operative Dentistry 2008;33(2):215–24.*

131. Odor TM, Chandler NP, Watson TF, et al. Laser light transmission in teeth: a study of the patterns in different species. *International Endodontic Journal* 1999;32:296–302.

132. Pioch T, Dushner H. Applications of Confocal laser scanning microscopy to dental bonding. *Adv Dent Res* 1997;11(4):453–61.

133. Perhavec T, Diaci J. Comparison of Er:YAG and Er, Cr:YSGG dental lasers. *J Oral Laser Applications* 2008;8:87–94.

134. Toshikazu Takeuchi, Koukichi Matsumoto. Application of lasers for treatment of pulp chamber perforations. *J Oral Laser Applications* 2008;8:225–34.

135. Ulrich Schoop, Wolf Kluger, Andreas Moritz. Bactericidal effect of different laser systems in the deep layers of dentin. *Lasers in Surgery and Medicine* 2004;35:111–16.

136. Ulrich Schoop, Kawe Goharkhay, Johannes Klimscha, Andreas Moritz. The use of erbium, chromium: yttrium-scandium-gallium-garnet laser in endodontic treatment: the results of an in vitro study. *JADA* 2007;139:949–55.

137. Gitirana VFD, Alves LP, Egberto Munin, et al. Study of the ablative effects of Nd:YAG or Er:YAG laser radiation. *Annals of Optics* 2003;5:1–3.

138. Walid Tawfik, Ali Saafan. Quantitative analysis of mercury in silver dental amalgam alloy using laser induced breakdown spectroscopy with a portable Echelle spectrometer. *International Journal of Pure and Applied Physics* 2006;2(3):195–203.

139. Wan-Hong Lan, Bor-Shiunn Lee. Morphologic study of Nd:YAG laser usage in treatment of dentinal hypersensitivity. *Journal of Endodontics* 2004;30(3):131–34.

140. Wolfgang Buchalla, Thomas Attin. External bleaching therapy with activation by heat, light or laser —a systematic review. *Dental Materials* 2007;23:586–96.

141. Yuichi Kimura, Wilder-Smith P, Koukichi Matsumoto. Lasers in endodontics: a review. *International Endodontic Journal* 2000;33:173–85.

142. Yuichi Kimura, Petra Wilder-Smith, Kazuo Yonago, Koukichi Matsumoto. Treatment of dentin hypersensitivity by lasers: a review. *J Clin Periodontol* 2000;27:715–21.

143. Zoran Karlovic, Sonja Pezelj-Ribaric. Erbium: YAG laser versus ultrasonic in preparation of root-end cavities. *JOE* 2005;31(11):821–23.

144. Adams TC, Pang PK. Lasers in aesthetic dentistry. *Dent Clin N Am* 48:2004:833–60.

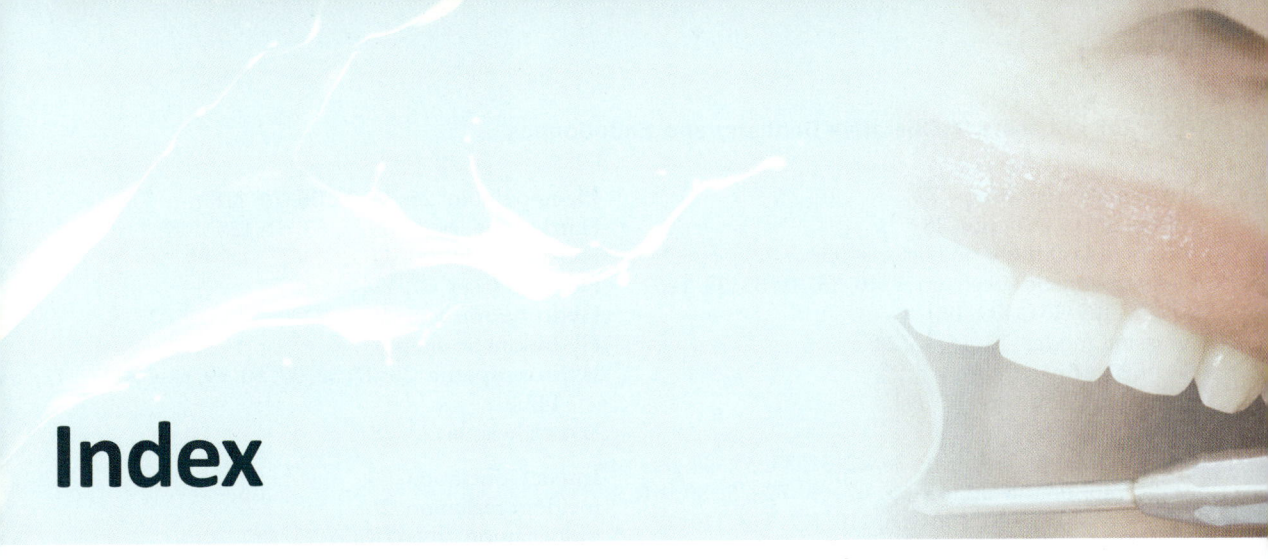

Index

Ablation 6, 28, 29, 32, 34, 36, 37, 59, 64, 66–68, 71–76, 95, 104, 138,145–148
Absorption 2, 26–29, 33–37, 42, 46, 52–53, 60, 64, 70, 73–76, 87, 93–97, 100–03, 109, 112, 118, 129, 138
Active medium 6–9, 14, 33–39, 130, 138–144
Aesthetic dentistry 150–51
Albert Einstein 2, 3, 8, 143
Alexandrite laser 35, 36,132
Amplification 1–3, 7, 9,138,141–43
Amplitude 7, 13, 14, 54, 158
Argon laser 29, 31, 35, 76–78, 91, 92,112, 119-21,126,131,138, 146–49
Arndt-Schultz law 84
Articulated arm 10, 11, 13, 28, 138, 143
Atomic clock 2
ATP 81, 87
Autoflourescence 41, 56
Average power 14, 36, 59, 107, 138, 143

Bacterial reduction
    with mid-infrared lasers 98
    with near-infrared lasers 97
Basic scheme of laser 8
Beam diameter 15, 16, 104,139
Beam profile 83,116
Bioresonance effect 72
Biostimulation 29,32,80,84
Brightness 16,76

Camphoroquinone 35, 76
Canary System™ 54–55
Cannula 22, 23
Carbonate 57, 64–67, 145
Caries 1, 6, 26–27, 30, 32, 34–48, 51–54, 59, 63, 65–68, 71, 74–76, 88, 92–93, 123, 129, 131–32, 145–50

Cataract formation 124, 126
Cavitation 41–2, 65, 96, 97, 103, 106, 109
Charles H. Townes 2–4
Chromophores 26, 27, 81
Cladding 19, 104, 139, 140
Cleave 19–22, 33, 105
Cluster probes 38, 81
CO_2 laser 11, 12, 33, 34, 63, 66, 67,72, 89, 92–95, 112, 113, 118, 126, 127, 129, 130, 131, 139
Coagulation 23, 24, 28, 30, 32, 37, 39, 40, 76, 93, 94, 112, 126, 129, 139
Coherence 1, 16, 41, 49–51,132, 139, 149
Cold lasers 80
Collimation 16, 17, 27, 139, 141
Confocal 55, 145, 147–150
Connes advantage 61
Contact mode 11, 15, 34, 35, 81, 139,142
Cooling system 8, 83, 135
Cosmetic resculpturing 116
Coupler 8, 19, 142
Crater 6, 63, 74, 116, 148
Crystal materials 62
Czerny–Turner monochromator 58

Defocused 15, 33, 34, 93, 117
DEKA 11, 69, 71,136
DIAGNOdent 41, 43–45, 68,145,148
Diamond 20, 62,149
Digital laser interferometry 78, 145
Diode laser 1, 18, 19, 22, 24, 32, 33, 38, 39, 52, 53, 55, 72, 75, 76, 82, 83, 89, 92, 96, 97, 99–103, 117–18, 130–39, 145, 148, 150
Directionality 8, 16, 17
Dose 63, 82, 84,101,133
Dye assisted laser ablation (DALA) 75

Earthquake sensations 72
Effects of laser energy 28
Effects of laser light on bacteria 95
Electromagnetic spectrum 9, 10, 16, 31, 33, 35, 126, 129, 131, 139, 140
Emission modes 13, 14, 18, 24
End-firing tips 97, 99
Endodontic retreatment 111
Endodontic tip 89, 98, 105
Energy 1,2, 7–9, 11–16, 19–20, 22–31, 33, 35, 37, 43, 46, 53, 58–60, 63–65, 67–69, 72–78, 80, 81, 84–87, 95–97, 100–108, 110, 112, 113, 119, 121, 126, 138–44
Energy density 15, 64, 67, 69, 74, 100, 101, 113, 140
Enterococcus faecalis 99, 100, 109
Er:YAG laser 37, 63–70, 72, 74, 89,90, 93, 98,99, 103, 107, 109, 111, 113, 150
Eschelle polychromator 58
Etching 32, 37, 56, 64, 103, 105, 106, 120
Excimer laser 5, 31, 72, 132, 140
Excitation mechanism 7
Eye injury 39, 124

Featherstone 34, 66, 131, 146, 148
Felgett advantage 61
Fiber cleaving 20
Fiberoptic delivery systems 22, 95, 103, 139
Fiber stripping 19
Fibroblasts 87, 94, 110
Fluence 15, 42, 67–69, 84, 86–88, 96, 103–06, 140
Focal plane array 52
Focusability 16, 17
Focused mode 116, 117
Focusing lens 8, 17, 140, 141
Fourier transform infrared spectroscopy 60, 62
Free running pulsed 23, 33, 36, 96, 132, 140
Free space electro-optical sampling 47
Frenectomy 33, 34, 36, 37, 71, 74, 75, 116, 117
Frequency 2,7, 9, 53-55, 59, 74, 75, 86, 88, 90, 93, 111, 118, 132, 140–43, 149
Fusobacterium nucleatum 99–102

GaAlAs (Gallium-aluminium-arsenide) laser 38, 39, 81, 92, 113
GaAs (gallium-arsenide) laser 14, 38, 51, 52, 143
Gain medium 7
Gaussian 96, 141, 144
Germanium 53, 62, 104, 105
Gingival troughing 33–37, 117–18
Goldman 6, 63

Haemoglobin 26, 33, 35, 36, 76, 118
Hard tissue laser 32, 37, 63, 64, 133, 148
Hibst and gall 43, 44
Ho:YAG laser 31, 124
Hydrofluoric acid 105
Hydrokinetic energy 75
Hydroxyapatite 26, 27, 32, 37, 50, 59, 64–66, 95, 112, 147
Hyperthermia 23, 28

Impact ionization 73
Incident radiation 26
Indocyanine green (ICG) 75, 100
Infrared laser 31, 64, 71, 72, 87, 95–98, 102, 103, 106, 138, 148
Infrared radiation 9, 60, 141
Infrared spectroscopy 60-62, 113, 146
InGaAlP (indium-gallium-aluminum-phosphide) laser 38, 81
Initiation 22, 40, 76
Intensity 2, 7, 15, 16, 37, 41, 45-49, 52, 53, 61, 80, 82, 91, 106, 119, 121, 128, 139, 141, 143, 144, 149
Internal reflection 12, 38, 104, 142
Ionizing 9, 36, 48, 59, 132, 141
Irradiance 14, 15, 75, 139, 141-144
Isotropic tips 105, 106

Knuckle 11

Laser ablation 72-75, 146, 148
Laser activated irrigation 96, 97, 102
Laser analgesia 71, 72, 148
Laser bleaching 118, 119, 121
Laser Doppler flowmetry 89, 90, 150
Laser fusion of dental casting alloys 78
Laser generated shock waves 103
Laser hazard classes 122
Laser holographic imaging 78
Laser induced breakdown spectroscopy (LIBS) 5, 57–59
Laser-modulated luminescence 41, 53
Laser photothermal radiometry 53, 55
Laser-powered hydrokinetic system (LPHKS) 69, 71
Laser safety officer 124, 128, 141
Laser toothbrush 88
Linear 78, 108, 145, 147

Mainman 129
MASER 2–4
Maxwell 2
Mirrors 7–11, 38, 53, 138, 141–43

Monochromatic 1, 9, 16, 22, 59, 76, 82, 139, 142, 142
Morikawa 89
Multi-radiance technology 87
Multi-photon imaging 45, 46

Neodymium 7, 31–33, 58, 63, 111, 112, 130, 131, 142
Near-infrared imaging 41, 52
Non-contact mode 11, 15, 35, 142
Nd:YAG laser 1, 5, 6, 10, 12, 16, 19, 23–27, 32,33, 36, 37, 58, 67, 71, 72, 89, 91–93, 96, 97, 103, 110–14, 116, 118, 124, 126, 129–33, 141, 142, 146–51

Optical coherence tomography 1, 41, 49, 50, 132, 149
Optical fiber 12, 14, 19, 33, 37, 38, 43, 50, 52, 58, 72, 76, 97, 104, 105, 142
Optical resonator 8, 138, 140, 142
Optical spectrum 9
Output coupler 8, 142

Pain 6, 18, 29, 30, 34, 39, 54, 63, 64, 67, 70–72, 75, 76, 80, 81, 84–92, 110, 120, 121, 128, 133
Peptostreptococcus micros 100
Photoacoustic 95, 97, 106–108, 111
Photoactivated disinfection 102, 106
Photochemical 29, 81, 95, 97, 103, 119
Photoelectric effect 2
Photomultiplier tube 55
Photon 2, 7–9, 17, 35, 37-39, 41, 43, 45–47, 54, 59, 64, 69, 77, 87, 97, 106, 107, 121, 131, 142, 143, 149
Photon-induced photoacoustic streaming (PIPS) 106–07
Photosensitizer molecules 99
Photothermal 22, 53, 55, 95, 97, 103, 107, 109
Planck's constant 2
Plasma-induced ablation 73
Plume 25, 72, 73, 126, 127, 142
Polarization 41, 50
Power 9, 10, 13–19, 23, 27–36, 38, 43, 46–48, 51, 55, 57–59, 63, 69, 73, 75–78, 80–83, 87, 89, 90, 91, 93, 95-97, 99, 101, 103, 104, 107, 108, 110, 111, 113, 120, 123, 125,130, 131, 133–35, 139–44, 147–48
Power density 14, 15, 19, 27, 58, 59, 77, 83, 103, 139, 141, 143
Prevotella intermedia 100, 102
Prism boundaries 66
Pulp capping 82, 92–94,111, 146, 147
Pulp chamber perforations 112, 150
Pulpitis 92

Pulpotomy 37, 89, 91–93,111
Pulse duration 13, 14, 33, 34, 58, 64, 67, 69, 72, 73, 95, 96, 104, 107, 110, 140, 143, 144
Pulsed 29, 30, 53, 58, 73, 120, 121, 124
Pumping mechanism 7, 33, 130, 140

Quantitative 41, 42, 61, 63, 145-150
Quantum 8, 73, 80, 142

Radial firing tip 97–99, 106, 111, 144
Radiation 1–3, 7, 9, 10, 13, 26, 34, 36, 43, 44, 47, 48, 53, 58–61, 64–68, 70, 72–75, 82, 84, 87, 90, 91, 95, 97–99, 101, 106, 109, 111–113, 122–28, 132, 138, 140–50
Raman spectroscopy 59, 60, 145, 147, 149
Rear mirror 8
Reflection 12, 27–29, 38, 48, 51, 64, 74, 89, 104, 123, 124, 126, 127, 142, 143
Repetition rate 13, 14, 69, 73, 141

Scattering 15, 28, 29, 42, 45–51, 54, 57, 59, 64, 93, 138
Semiconductor lasers 4, 5, 38, 143
Signal averaging 61
Smile 115
Smoke evacuation 126, 127
Sodium hypochlorite 102–5, 107, 109
Soft-tissue lasers 23, 32, 37
Solid-state lasers 14, 73, 130
Spectral encoding 60
Spontaneous emission 3, 8, 143
Static magnetic field 87
Stern and sognnaes 63
Stimulated emission 1–3, 5, 7–9, 17, 38, 138, 141, 143
Streptococcus 102
Superluminescent diodes 52
Super-pulsed 13, 14, 87, 93
Sweep 83

Terahertz 41, 47-49, 131, 146, 147
Thermal relaxation time 96, 143, 144
Tips 12, 44, 45, 75, 83, 87, 89, 96–99, 104, 111, 139
Tolonium chloride 100, 101
Total internal reflection 12, 104
Transmission 12, 27, 29, 38, 43, 48, 52, 60, 64, 72, 98, 103–6, 144, 147, 150
Tricalcium phosphate 112
Turbulent 108
Twinlight endodontic treatment 110, 111

Ultra-short pulse laser ablation 73
Ultraviolet 10

Vaporization 22, 28, 30, 32, 33, 37, 65, 66, 74, 86, 138, 140, 144

Visible light 9, 10, 31, 77, 80, 81, 82, 123, 138, 142

Waterlase 75, 148
Waveguides 11- 13
Wavelength 2, 4–12, 14, 16, 26-39, 41, 43, 44, 46, 47,
        49, 53, 55, 58, 61, 63, 64, 66, 67, 69, 73–77, 80–
        95, 97, 100, 103–05, 107, 109–14, 118 121,
        124, 126–35, 138–40, 142, 144, 147

Weichman and Johnson 89
Welded 28, 79

Xenon 5, 34, 41, 132, 142

Young's experiment 2

Zinc selenide 62
Zur Theorie der Strahlung 2